the**facts**

Back pain

JOHN LEE
Pain Management Centre

National Hospital for Neurology and Neurosurgery,
London

SUZANNE BROOK
Pain Management Centre

National Hospital for Neurology and Neurosurgery,
London

CLARE DANIEL
Pain Management Centre

National Hospital for Neurology and Neurosurgery,
London;

NHS Islington GP Direct Access Physiotherapy Service,
London

OXFORD
UNIVERSITY PRESS

OXFORD

UNIVERSITY PRESS

Great Clarendon Street, Oxford OX2 6DP

Oxford University Press is a department of the University of Oxford.
It furthers the University's objective of excellence in research, scholarship,
and education by publishing worldwide in

Oxford New York

Auckland Cape Town Dar es Salaam Hong Kong Karachi
Kuala Lumpur Madrid Melbourne Mexico City Nairobi
New Delhi Shanghai Taipei Toronto

With offices in

Argentina Austria Brazil Chile Czech Republic France Greece
Guatemala Hungary Italy Japan Poland Portugal Singapore
South Korea Switzerland Thailand Turkey Ukraine Vietnam

Oxford is a registered trade mark of Oxford University Press
in the UK and in certain other countries

Published in the United States
by Oxford University Press Inc., New York

© Oxford University Press 2009

The moral rights of the authors have been asserted
Database right Oxford University Press (maker)

First edition published 2009

British Library Cataloguing in Publication Data

Data available

Library of Congress Cataloging in Publication Data

Lee, John, 1963-
    Back pain / John Lee, Suzanne Brook, Clare Daniel. — 1st ed.
      p. cm. — (The facts)
    Includes index.
    ISBN 978-0-19-956107-0
    1. Backache—Popular works. I. Brook, Suzanne, 1967- II. Daniel, Clare,
1966-. III. Title
    RD771.B217L44 2009
    617.5'64—dc22

                                                    2009013182

Typeset in Plantin
by Cepha Imaging Pvt. Ltd., Bangalore, India
Printed in Great Britain by Ashford Colour Press Ltd, Gosport, Hampshire

ISBN 978-0-19-9561-070

10 9 8 7 6 5 4 3 2 1

Preface

Back pain is a common condition: 70 per cent of people have back pain at some time or other. In each month, one in eight people aged between 16 and 64 years old are not at work because of back pain. These are pretty staggering figures and scientific studies have looked at the costs to the UK of back pain. When you take into account not only the health costs (tablets, NHS attendances, private osteopathy, acupuncture and so on) but also the indirect costs (for example government benefits, lost tax to the government, or lost earnings because a loved one has to give up work to look after the person with pain) the amount spent on back pain in the UK is more than 20 per cent of the total NHS budget. In today's terms, this is around £16 billion (equivalent to US$ 23,000,000,000), a phenomenal amount of money. Back pain is so prevalent that it is the subject of national and multinational guidance in the UK, Europe, the United States, Australia and New Zealand. In the UK, the National Institute for Health and Clinical Excellence (NICE) is producing guidelines for people with chronic back pain (2009).

As a common condition, people can often become blasé about it. However, back pain can be so disabling and pervasive that to not pay proper attention to it is a mistake. This book has been written to help people take more control of their own back pain. It does this in three different ways:

1 it explains why back pain can develop

2 it shows what medical treatments are available and which are likely to be more successful than others

3 it describes ways to help yourself both with the doctor's guidance and independently.

For many people with back pain there is no quick fix solution, but there are ways to make sure you live life as fully as possible receiving the best options in healthcare and taking all the opportunities available from the gift of life.

Throughout the book there are multiple examples and patients' tales of their situation. No two people are ever the same but the prevalence of back pain means that it has been the subject of a large number of medical studies. The guidance in this book comes from many decades of collecting knowledge about back pain as well as the invaluable experience of three clinicians with a wealth of experience in this group of patients. The book should empower the individual with the knowledge to find the best course of action for them.

Contents

Section 4

Bringing things together and real patients' stories

Section 1

Understanding back pain

1

How is the back constructed?

➡ Key Points

- The human back is part of the unique skeleton that distinguishes our species from most animals
- We are born to live life upright and the back gives structure and mechanical support to allow this
- Strong muscles, tendons and ligaments all work together with the spinal column to form the human back
- It is designed to be flexible, to carry weight and to move in a large number of directions
- Our back connects our head and arms to our pelvis and legs which together make up our body: a major accomplishment of bioengineering

Introduction

The spine is made up of a series of similar bones lying on top of each other, called vertebrae. Not only does the spine provide flexible structural support to the body, it also protects the spinal cord, which is the major bundle of nerves travelling to and from the brain to the trunk and limbs. It does this because each vertebra contains a ring structure and when all the vertebrae are added together, a pipe is formed from the aligned rings. The soft nervous tissue of the spinal cord is thus afforded the same level of protection as the brain, which is housed in the solid bony structure of the skull. However, the spine is required to be flexible and allow access for passing nerves, so at each spinal level there are paired passages and gaps.

Anatomy of the vertebrae and intervertebral discs

The spine, or vertebral column, has 24 vertebrae (Figure 1.1). There are:

- seven neck (cervical) vertebrae
- twelve chest (thoracic) vertebrae and
- five lower back (lumbar) vertebrae.

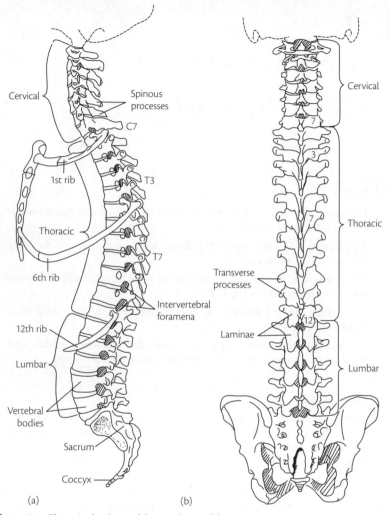

Figure 1.1 The spinal column. (a) Lateral view, (b) Posterior view.

The lumbar vertebrae join the sacrum which is in fact a fusion of five sacral vertebrae to form one solid and strong bone. The sacrum transfers much of the upper body's weight to the pelvis and legs through a large, strong joint at the base of the spine, the sacroiliac joint. The sacrum forms part of the ring of the pelvis, which supports our internal organs, and it is one of the most rigid sections of our body.

The coccyx is the last bony part of the vertebral column; if we had a tail, this is what we would wag. Medical terminology often describes each vertebra by a letter and a number where the letter stands for the section of the spine and the number for the individual vertebra, counting down from the head. So, C5 would refer to the fifth cervical vertebra counting from the top down, and L5 refers to the fifth lumbar vertebra which connects to the sacrum.

> My doctor keeps talking about the joints of my back and my discs. I really haven't a clue what she is talking about. I thought the back was a fairly rigid and strong structure?

Doctors may use the following terms when explaining your back problem to you. Although each vertebra is one single bone, it has channels, grooves and surfaces which are designed to touch other surfaces (see Figure 1.2).

- *Vertebral body.* The largest part of each bone is the vertebral body and this bears most of the weight that the spine supports. It is the front part of any vertebra. In medical terms, the front is towards the nose or belly button and is called *anterior*, with the opposite direction being called *posterior*.

- *Pedicles.* Behind the vertebral body are paired pedicles (left- and right-sided). The pedicles are not as tall as the vertebral bodies and have a curved notch on their upper and lower surfaces.

- *Foramen.* The notches on the pedicles form a foramen (the Latin word for a hole) on the left and right sides through which the spinal nerves can leave the spinal canal.

- *Transverse processes.* The pedicles give off transverse processes on both sides.

- *Laminae.* The transverse processes become the laminae as they run posteriorly.

- *Facet joints.* As the laminae move posteriorly, they then give rise to the facet joints (also called zygoapophyseal joints) which connect with the vertebra above and below.

- *Spinous process.* The laminae come together posteriorly to form the single midline spinous process which is the part of the spine that is easy to feel in the midline on your back.

As mentioned above, the vertebrae connect with their neighbours through the paired facet joints. These joints are synovial joints (like the knee or finger joints) which means they allow movement between the surfaces they connect with. They do this because the moving surfaces are covered with cartilage (articular cartilage) and the whole joint (i.e. the moving surfaces of the vertebra above and below) has a capsule around it filled with very slippery fluid (synovial fluid).

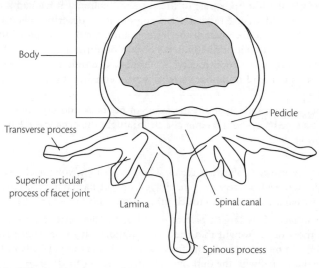

Figure 1.2 A life-sized lumbar vertebra.

The vertebrae also connect through the intervertebral discs, each of which has:

* a tough outer ring called an annulus fibrosis, and

* a softer jelly-like interior called the nucleus pulposus (see Figure 1.4).

The intervertebral discs are around one centimetre high and follow the contours of the end plates of the vertebral bodies they are next to. It works very well to call them the 'shock absorbers' of the spine because they can be compressed when the vertebrae are forced together (like when landing from a jump, or bending) and go back to their normal shape when this extra force has stopped.

Nerve supplies to the body and limbs

The nerves travel down from the brain as the spinal cord and give off left and right pairs of spinal nerves at each vertebral level which then pass through the paired intervertebral foraminae.

The nerves send messages to provide muscle control and receive messages about pain, temperature, vibration, the position of the joints (e.g. bent or straight) and so on. The spinal cord gets progressively thinner as it gives off its nerves. At around the level of the first lumbar vertebra, the spinal cord comes to an end and the remaining nerves run down inside the spinal canal clumped together as the cauda equina (again Latin, for horse's tail).

The nerves flow out from the spinal cord in a sequence from top to bottom with the arms being supplied first by nerves in the neck (cervical region), then the

torso (thoracic region), followed by the legs and lastly, the genitals, anus and rec-
tum (lumbar and sacral region). The passage of these nerves is well understood
and we know the territory of skin that is served by each paired spinal nerve. We
call the area of skin supplied by one spinal nerve a *dermatome* (see Figure 1.3).

However, it should be remembered that spinal nerves often join together after
they have left the spinal column and combine to form larger nerves. One example of this is the largest nerve in the body, the sciatic nerve which is formed
from the fourth lumbar nerve (L4) along with L5; and first sciatic nerve (S1)
along with S2 and S3.

Spinal movement and strength

The bones that make up the spine are supported by ligaments (very tough
restraining tissue that joins bones to other bones). Ligaments are like a piece of

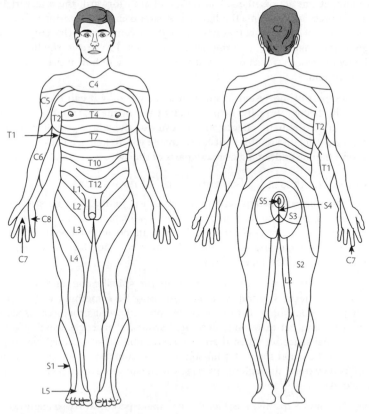

Figure 1.3 Body dermatomes.

rope tethering a ship to the dock allowing shortening but not much lengthening. They are also supported by muscles and their tendons (tendons connect muscles to bones). Without these, the spine would not be able to do much of its job. The ligaments, muscles and tendons work together, not only to enable the spine to move, but also to provide a lot of structural strength.

The nerves send messages about how muscles should contract (most of which is automatic and not at a conscious level) and receive messages about the state of tension these structures are in. Looking at the back's structure, the head articulates on the spine, the spine transmits force through the pelvis to the hips, the whole complex is held together by incredibly strong tendons, muscles and ligaments, and the nerves transmit messages to and from the system to 'read' the current state and to send messages for movement.

The body is designed for movement and its parts have enough 'give' to allow the most flexible of us to reach forward and touch the floor with our hands. If we look at this action, the spinal bones all arch forward, the intervertebral discs compress at the front, the ligaments extend in the posterior part of the spine, the spinal cord and nerves have enough movement and elasticity to allow a significant lengthening, and the hands can reach forward to the floor. This flexibility reduces as we get older, but it gives an idea of how much 'give' there is in the system.

If any one part of the system is not working as best as it can then the whole complex is affected. Equally, helping many parts of the system in a small way can have quite dramatic effects on the result of the whole complex. In later chapters we will build on this concept to enable you to manage back pain better by reconditioning and toning as many parts of the system as possible.

Alphabetical glossary of common spinal conditions

Arthritis this literally means 'inflammation of the joints'. The most common form is osteoarthritis and the numbers of people affected rise with age. It is from a process of wearing or degeneration. It often affects multiple joints including the knees, hips hands and spine and is the most common form of disability of older people in the developed world.

Canal stenosis the 'canal' referred to means the spinal canal, and this can be narrow, or stenotic. Central canal stenosis may be something you are born with, i.e. it is congenital. It can also come on with wear processes, especially when facet joints get extra bone deposited around their edges which protrude into the canal space, or when there is intervertebral disc material which protrudes into the canal space. Canal stenosis can sometimes cause pinching of nerves as they travel through the passage which can give rise to pain, numbness or weakness.

Degenerate or degenerative these terms often make people worry so many doctors now choose other words instead. However, they remain in common medical use.

They mean a process of wear which comes on with age. It is not possible to turn the clock back on the ageing process and our body changes as we get older. Signs of wear can appear from teenage years onwards.

Dehydrated disc as we know, dehydrated means to have less water content. A dehydrated disc is one which shows less water content when compared with a healthy disc. A dehydrated disc will not be as tall as a healthy one and when visualized with an MRI scan, the reduced water content shows clearly. This sort of dehydration does not relate to overall body hydration. It is another sign of wear which often comes on with age and is one of the reasons that people get shorter as they get older.

Foraminal stenosis in many ways this is similar to canal stenosis, but it relates to the paired intervertebral foraminae which allow nerves to leave the spinal canal between each vertebral bone. If facet joints deposit extra bone around the intervertebral foramen, or if there is some intervertebral disc material protruding towards the foramen, the foramen may developing a narrowing or stenosis, leading to pinching of the nerves as they travel through. This might affect the right or the left sides.

Oedema oedema means swelling: this means is that there is an increase in the amount of fluid in something. In terms of the spine, occasionally there are signs of oedema when a wear or degenerative process is active. As with many observations seen on a magnetic resonance imaging (MRI) scan, there is no means of intervening to change this.

Prolapsed disc this term is used a lot with reference to back pain, leg pain and sciatica. The reason for this is that it is both a frequent finding on scans and a common event. A bit of intervertebral disc material bulges backward from its normal confines and protrudes into the central canal or an intervertebral foramen (Figure 1.4). Disc material usually prolapses to the rear (towards your back not your front) because this is where the pressure is transmitted when bending forwards. This material can favour one side or the other, or it can be more diffuse.

Slipped, protruding, ruptured or torn disc a 'slipped' disc is really a misnomer. It suggests something that has travelled some way. It really means a prolapsed disc (see above). Some patients have reported that they imagined the disc has slipped to travel somewhere it shouldn't be, which reflects how misleading the term slipped disc can be. Most often, a slipped disc refers to a bulge of an intervertebral disc into the central spinal canal, and usually with no adverse effects or symptoms. A protruding disc is very similar.

Some doctors use a variety of similar terms to mean the same thing, but in different degrees; some might say a protrusion is bigger than a bulge, but it is clear to see that these terms can be so similar that they become confusing, even for the medical staff. When the terms 'ruptured' or 'torn' or 'herniated' are used, this means that the disc capsule has given way and some of the inner contents

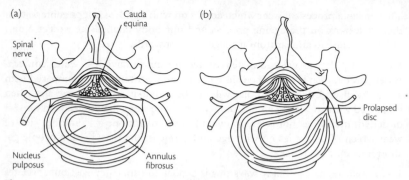

Figure 1.4 An intervertebral disc prolapse. (a) Lumbar intervertebral disc viewed from below, (b) prolapse of nucleus pulposus (slipped disc).

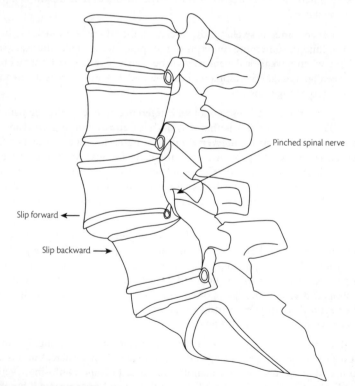

Figure 1.5 Spondylolisthesis.

are exposed. The body will endeavour to repair the damage. The contents can cause irritation and inflammation around the area which can lead to pain and muscle spasm.

Schmorl's nodes these are protrusions of intervertebral disc material into the vertebral body above or below. They are sometimes seen on X-ray and will also be detected by an MRI scan. They are associated with wear of the spine. It is not entirely clear why they form or what their role is in relation to pain. At the moment, they are a marker of wear of the spine and little else.

Sciatica sciatica means pain in the distribution of the sciatic nerve. This nerve is made up of the nerve roots from L4, L5, S1, S2 and S3 with pain felt in the lower back, buttock, or the lower leg and foot. There are left and right sides of this nerve and it is the largest nerve in the body. Although sciatica may come from different causes, it is often from irritation of a nerve in the back. It is sometimes associated with pins and needles in the same distribution, or weakness of the muscles.

Spondylolisthesis this complex word is the slippage of one vertebra relative to another (Figure 1.5). It is often seen where people have wear or degeneration of the spine. It may be reported in percentage terms (e.g. 25 per cent slippage of one vertebra over another) or in four stages where stage 1 = up to 25 per cent slippage, stage 2 = 25 to 50 per cent slippage and so on. It can give rise to symptoms if nerves are pinched by the process or if there is a lot of movement of one bone over another.

Spondylosis spondylosis is wear or degeneration of the spine and is a general term relating to the multiple parts that make up the spine.

2

What is back pain?

➲ Key Points

- Understanding your pain can be the key to tackling it
- There are fundamental differences between acute pain and long-term pain
- In long-term back pain, the link between damage and pain is often not very clear
- Having back pain not only affects your body but how you manage your life and relationships with others

Introduction

The question 'what is back pain?' is understandable but the answer can be complicated. This chapter discusses:

- why people feel pain at all
- the difference between acute and long-term pain
- how the body repairs itself
- how pathways can develop that promote long-term back pain.

It also describes the definitions of pain used both in everyday life and in scientific literature which demonstrate how pain affects us in so many different ways. Understanding the origins of a problem usually go a long way to managing them better.

📄 Case study Part 1

Charles did not understand why he had pain that would not go away. In school he played rugby and cricket. He was a good cross country runner. He continued rugby at university. In his early twenties, he started to have back pain which would be particularly problematic when he had to sit for a long time in lectures. He decided to try and seek some help and, after a few medical consultations, he underwent an operation to his lumbar spine where two of the vertebrae were fused together. He was very pleased with the results as his back pain was much better. However, after about a year, the same symptoms started creeping back. Pain when standing too long, sitting too long, and when he tried to go running to keep fit.

Why do I have pain?

Pain is a biological development so that more complex organisms can react to protect themselves from a threat. As an example, some creatures that are made of only one single cell respond to touch, temperature or changing environment by moving away. Humans are one of the most highly developed biological creatures. We not only react rapidly to unpleasant stimuli (like withdrawing our hand by reflex when we accidentally touch something very hot) but also learn behaviour based on our past experiences.

Acute pain and the repair process

Pain itself can be separated broadly into two types:

1 *acute pain*—pain that is short lived and from which you are likely to recover

2 *chronic* or *long-term pain*—pain that goes on for a long time.

Acute pain occurs in response to a tissue injury where there is usually tissue damage and associated inflammation, followed by a process of repair and healing that lasts for days or months. The inflammation may or may not be visible. Chemical signals, transmitters, specialized cells, nerves and receptors are all involved in the system which is there to warn of danger and then protect injured parts until they have been put back together as best as the body is able.

In the back, an acute pain may arise from a torn muscle or intervertebral disc. The body will sense damaged cells because the inside contents of cells are released ; other monitoring cells which travel throughout the body pick up this and 'swarm' to the damaged area to start the process of repair. Swelling and tightness often occur as the local fluid levels change with more water in the area than normal (oedema or swelling). Local acidity levels and local oxygen levels may also change. The nerves will sense all these changes and have local responses in controlling blood flow as well as sending messages to the spinal cord and the brain to increase the protection of the damaged area at a reflex and a conscious level.

Depending on the size of the injury, this healing process may take a few days to a few months, but in most cases, by six months healing is complete and tissues have remodelled themselves. This whole process is aided by movement, exercise and returning to normal activities.

The origins of long-term pain

Long-term pain often starts with an episode of acute pain; there may be an injury just like that described above. The process of repair will start and complete, but pain persists for months or years after the triggering event. We now understand that this is not a helpful process; it is likely to be a fault in the nervous system that promotes continuing pain rather than healing. Messages about pain are being transmitted even though there is no ongoing damage that needs to be repaired or danger that needs to be protected, for example an oversensitive alarm that is ringing and ringing although there is no crime in progress.

A lot of scientific study is trying to discover why this process happens, to see if there are ways of avoiding it. There are a number of changes that we know occur in the nerves travelling to the limbs and trunk, the nerves that join up with other nerves within the spinal cord, the nerves that process messages in the brain, the absolute numbers of nerves involved, and the nerves that send messages back to the spinal cord to control feedback mechanisms. So far, medicine is not very good at changing the way nerves promote long-term pain, but a better understanding of the mechanisms may lead to future discoveries of new drugs and other treatments.

> Long-term pain is likely to be a fault in the nervous system that promotes continuing pain rather than healing. Messages about pain are being transmitted even though there is no ongoing damage.

Definitions of pain

There is a textbook definition of pain used by the International Association for the Study of Pain which is widely quoted: 'an unpleasant sensory and emotional experience associated with actual or potential tissue damage, or described in terms of such damage'. Although this uses rather scientific terms, it is a useful definition and there are some key features to look at more carefully:

♦ it is accepted that pain causes an emotional experience as well as a sensory one;

♦ actual tissue damage may not be evident; and

♦ the link between damage and pain may not be strong, i.e. it is only described as an association.

This last point is interesting and important. In long-term back pain, the link between damage and pain is often not very clear. This is because the changes in the nervous system have amplified the pain and caused it to be a persistent problem, even though the injury or damage has long since healed.

People's descriptions of pain

When people are asked to describe pain, they often struggle both because it can be described in so many ways and because it is very hard to put the experience into words. The experience of pain also changes depending on the time of day, whether you are hot or cold, your mood and what you are doing at the time. As a result, there is a plethora of words to describe pain and none of these are wrong.

Doctors often ask you to describe your pain as sometimes the answers you give help them consider certain structures that may be the cause. The terms 'burning', 'tingling', 'electric' or 'itchy' can mean that there is nerve damage in the area of pain; 'tightness', 'aching' or 'weakness' can describe muscle pain. Other words describe how your pain makes you feel. The most important thing for you to remember is that these are descriptive words and they are not always linked to what has happened. They are all helpful in understanding how the pain affects you.

It is also the case that people are unable to describe their pain. In the text box is what looks like a jumble of words. They are in fact all words which have been used by people to describe their pain. It demonstrates how pain affects people at physical, emotional and sensory levels.

Words people use to decribe their pain

Excruciating nagging nauseating discomforting distressing horrible agonizing dreadful torturing annoying troublesome miserable intense unbearable spreading radiating penetrating piercing tight numb drawing squeezing tearing cool cold freezing suffocating fearful frightful annoying electric buzzing cruel vicious killing wretched blinding itchy smarting stinging dull sore hurting aching heavy tender mild taut rasping splitting tiring exhausting sickening pinching pressing gnawing cramping crushing tugging pulling wrenching hot boring scalding searing tingling flickering quivering pulsing throbbing beating pounding jumping flashing shooting pricking boring drilling stabbing lancinating sharp cutting lacerating

---

Back pain encompasses more than just the muscles, joints and nerves

When you begin to describe back pain in full, it is not just physical things that come out in the description; your back pain is not just about your back but about the whole of you. Clinicians who work in this field have a special term for this and call it the *biopsychosocial* model (see Table 2.1). Needless to say:

◆ *bio* refers to biological aspects of pain

◆ *psycho* the influence of psychology on pain experiences, and

◆ *social* is the aspect of pain where the sufferer interacts with the people around in society.

Focusing on any one aspect of the *bio*, *psycho* and *social* may not lead to as effective an improvement as if you can think about all three of its parts.

Tackling back pain effectively means:

◆ understanding how your back works

◆ considering the treatments and medications that might help

◆ improving movement, exercise and stretch levels

◆ tackling unhelpful thoughts and feelings

◆ making sure that your own situation is as good as it can be to help you move forward (in the home, at work or out and about).

These issues are developed further throughout this book.

Why do some people seem to experience pain differently to others?

The simplest answer to this question is that everyone is different. Men and women feel pain a little differently. In some cultures, the number of people

Table 2.1 The biopsychosocial model of pain

Biopsychosocial model of pain	Examples of effects
Bio	I find standing in a queue painful
	I used to love exercising regularly but now it just hurts
	I can't go on holiday because of all the sitting needed to get there
Psycho	I worry that I will damage my back by exercise
	I am frightened my back will break
	I get so depressed when I can't play with my youngest child
Social	My friends don't understand why I don't go out any more
	I had to give up work because my work as a telephonist needed me to sit for too long
	I used to bring in a decent salary and now I am dependent on my partner and benefits

complaining of long-term pain is different from others. There are also major genetic problems that mean that there are a few families of people that feel no pain at all. This gives rise to its own problems as people often end up being seriously injured because they do not realize they have been hurt.

There are also social differences amongst those who feel pain. People who are self-employed appear to report less pain that those who work for an employer. We also know that people who are busy with regular jobs fare better than people who are not. All of these differences are interesting as they raise questions: answering the questions can lead to potentials for helping people.

📄 Case study Part 2

At the same time that Charles' pain began to come back after surgery, he had moved and started work as a junior producer for the BBC. He had begun struggling at work as he had to sit for long periods of time working on computers. His new GP advised him to attend a local pain clinic. At the clinic he received more advice about his back pain which enabled him both to better understand his condition and to make plans he was happy with. He worked towards increasing the exercise he could tolerate and he also found he was better able to manage his working life. His general happiness was much improved.

Bringing the components of long-term pain together

Many people, including some medical staff and clinicians, focus on one part of the body, often on the things that can be seen on a scan or an X-ray. However, medicine alone often cannot fix the reasons for developing long-term pain because the roots of the problem are related to medical, psychological and social issues and each aspect needs attention. Additionally, medicine is not able to refashion or restructure nervous systems that have adapted to a way of working that incorporates long-term pain at the level of cells or the connections between nerve cells.

In long-term pain, vicious cycles are often found where a small problem becomes magnified and maintained. Added to these there may be additional pressures that make the whole situation worse, such as:

◆ being unable to work leads to pressure from an employer

◆ a reduced income leads to pressures at home

◆ employment problems will also lead to social consequences (e.g. the roles at home, or perceptions amongst wider family and friends)

* income, employment and social problems will lead to an effect on mood
* a low mood can worsen the experience of pain.

Long-term pain is a major health issue because so many people in the world have it. In a number of countries whose healthcare systems are similar, around 20 per cent of the population suffers long-term pain with a slight preponderance of women. Governments, everyone involved in healthcare and people with back pain would be pleased if those who might be at risk of getting long-term pain could be targeted effectively in an early stage to help them learn improved techniques for managing their situation. The right way to address long-term back pain is by using an holistic approach which is backed up by both experience and scientific evidence.

3

Scans, X-rays and that word 'degenerating'

➲ Key Points

♦ As with the rest of our bodies, the spine changes with time and these changes can be seen on X-rays and MRI scans

♦ For most people with back pain, there is no need to have an X-ray or scan because this will not change the advice or treatment you are given

♦ Many people with changes on their X-rays or scans have never had back pain

♦ Movement, activity and stretching are all excellent ways of looking after your musculoskeletal system as time goes on

There are very few of us who do not have parts of our bodies which at some time we wished looked different. Our spines are the same in that they often do not look like the textbook descriptions. In addition, our spines get older as time goes on, just like the rest of our body. This is a natural process which also happens to our hair, skin, nails, teeth, eyes, ears, bones, joints, muscles and internal organs. Chapter 1 largely described the spine without any signs of ageing. This chapter will talk more about the ageing process and the scans that can reveal it.

The spine as time goes on

As far as bone density is concerned, from around the age of 30 we all lose a little bit of bone density each year. Women suffer from this more than men as the female hormone oestrogen helps to protect from bone loss and the production of this hormone decreases after women enter the menopause. Bone modelling occurs where the natural repair cycle of bones leads to new bone formation. As part of this cycle, new bone production is influenced by mechanical stresses which can change the shape of bones like the vertebrae, as well as add spurs of bones (osteophytes) around the edges of bones and joints to help spread the load.

As the spine ages, its bone density decreases and it is less able to withstand the forces that it did in young adult life. Fractures can occur in the vertebrae just as they often happen in the wrists or hips of older people. The ligaments and muscles supporting the bones and joints can also weaken and result in one bone shifting position in relationship to another, as seen in spondylolisthesis (see Chapter 1 for an explanation of this and many other terms).

The intervertebral discs are also subject to ageing. Typically their water content decreases and they become relatively dehydrated compared to their pristine condition in youth. This sort of dehydration is not because of whole body dehydration and cannot be corrected by drinking; it is just a change with time and is combined with a decrease in the spongy elasticity of the disc. One of the results of this process can be that a prolapsed intervertebral disc occurs. This in itself is a relatively minor event and happens often with no symptoms for the individual. The side wall of the disc bulges a little outwards and often backwards; humans most often put their discs under strain when they bend forwards: this puts pressure on the front of the disc which is transmitted to the rear disc wall. A prolapsed intervertebral disc is a colourful medical term which sounds much worse than what it is in reality—a sag in the side wall of a tough structure.

What is the difference between a scan, an X-ray and a CT or MRI?

A 'scan' is a crude term that means some sort of imaging. There are different ways to image the body, and the word scan could mean any of them. It is a widely used term but it is not very accurate.

An X-ray shines X-ray radiation at the body, and shadows are cast depending on the different densities of the parts of the body. The images are captured on X-ray film or a digital receiver. More solid parts of the body (like bones) absorb more of the X-rays than the less solid parts (like the lungs); in this way an image is created. It is a very useful tool but it is not possible to see fine details.

A CT scan takes multiple X-ray pictures in one sitting and a high powered computer processes the results to produce exceedingly detailed pictures. CT stands for computerized tomography, and a CT scanner is able to piece together lots of more coarse images to get very refined ones. However, in doing so it uses a lot of radiation.

A magnetic resonance imaging (MRI) scan uses different technology where the part of the body to be examined is placed in an exceedingly high magnetic field which makes the molecules of the body line up in one direction. The magnetic field is then relaxed and the molecules 'wobble' as they go back to random movements. When they do this, they emit different electromagnetic radiation depending on the tissues they are made up of. Again, this process is repeated multiple times to create composite images of the body.

In general terms, X-rays are better at looking at things which are more solid (like spinal bones) and MRI scans are better at looking at things with higher water content (like the brain, nerves and the softer structures around joints like cartilage and synovium). A lateral MRI of the spine is shown in Figure 3.1.

If a prolapsed disc is going to give rise to symptoms, a frequent presentation is when the disc protrudes around the intervertebral foramen because at this point the spinal nerve is travelling out from the spinal canal to the structures it supplies, for example the legs or arms. The hole it travels through is very close to the intervertebral discs and the nerve is vulnerable to being pinched if the disc bulges into its path. This can give rise to pain, pins and needles or numbness in the region supplied by a nerve, so if the first sacral nerve (S1) is pinched, the symptoms will be felt deep in the buttock and down the back of the leg. The nervous supply to the body was mapped out many centuries ago, but like the rest of the body it does not always exactly match the textbooks—humans vary quite a bit from one person to the next!

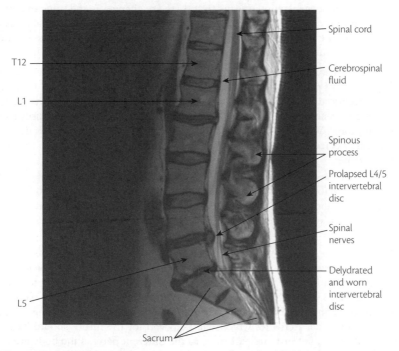

Figure 3.1 An MRI scan of the lumbar spine, seen from the side. Note how structures with a high water content (such as cerebrospinal fluid and intervertebral discs) show as a lighter shade.

For most people with simple back pain, there is no need to have an X-ray or a scan because scientific evidence shows us that having the images does not change the medical outcomes. It is possible that it can do harm, too, because it can make people focus on parts of the back rather than thinking about the whole solution to the problem which involves increased movement, stretching, and returning to normal activities. Images are helpful if you have nerve symptoms to check the cause because unlike bone, nerves do not regenerate very well.

Degeneration and what can be done about it

There are two factors that determine how imaging of our spine shows differences from the textbook of perfection:

◆ the way we are designed, and

◆ the modelling that occurs as part of the ageing process.

Many reports of X-rays and MRI scans talk about 'degeneration' because this is a medical term in regular use to describe changes related to the aging process. The term 'degeneration' means that there are changes in the spine that are the result of the normal process of ageing. It is used to distinguish the changes from those due to some other process such as changes due to a broken bone (fracture) or due to an infection.

In a medical study published in the *Annals of Internal Medicine* in 2002, up to 81 per cent of people who had no symptoms of back or leg pain had bulging intervertebral discs, up to 93 per cent of people who had degenerative discs also had no pain and up to 56 per cent of people with a tear in their discs had no symptoms. What this shows us is that changes that are seen on scans do not necessarily correlate with the symptoms you have and that you have to put the two together.

> Scientists have performed MRI scans on normal people who have no back symptoms and no back pain and have found some to have slipped intervertebral discs, signs of ageing of the discs, or tears in their discs.

Keeping active, moving and stretching joints, ligaments and tendons, and giving your nerves information to work on within the normal range of movements are all ways to improve the function of the spinal complex (see Chapter 11). These are also ways of making it less likely that you will have future damage to your body and spine. However, it is not possible to counteract ageing which happens to us all. Activities which will help you for the future should be for the whole body, not just one part of it, as the different parts of the body are all interrelated with one another. Scientific evidence provides a lot of good-quality support for this global approach to self-help.

4

How did the pain get to take over my life?

⊃ Key Points

- It is not easy living with, and managing, pain
- Pain can affect your life in many different ways, and vary from person to person
- It is not your fault that previous treatments have not made the pain go away
- It can often feel like a downward spiral but by using pain management strategies you can gain more control of your pain

Some people who have long-term pain can identify exactly when their pain started; others say that it just gradually crept up on them and seemed to start for no apparent reason. Whatever the reason, everyone tries their hardest to make it go away. Some of the things that people try can be helpful initially but in the long term they can lose their effect and eventually become more unhelpful than helpful. At these times people often think it is their fault that treatments and therapies do not work but as you will have already read, pain changes the longer you have had it and the approach to managing and treating your pain needs to change too.

When someone has pain it can begin to take over many areas of their life. Whether you have had pain for a day or a year, pain can affect people in different ways. If you think of all the things that pain has affected in your day-to-day life, the length of the list may surprise you. Below are some of the things that people with pain have told us about.

1 *Mobility (e.g. walking)*—people commonly say that, over time, they are able to do less. Walking to the bus stop becomes harder and because of that it is done less often. Taking the stairs at the train station or at work become less frequent; you use the lift instead. Some of you may start to use a stick, thinking it may help your mobility, but long term you may wonder if this makes things worse.

2 *Mood (e.g. depression, anger, frustration, and anxiety)*—it is understandable that if any area of your life is affected by pain there may be some effect on your mood. Many people feel that since the pain

started, feelings of low mood have become significant and this has a knock-on effect on other areas of life—a vicious cycle has started.

3 *Family*—having pain all the time can affect the way you interact with those around you or react to those you care about and love. You may find you are snappy and find it hard to listen to others or that they may appear unsympathetic to your pain.

4 *Fitness*—many people have stopped doing exercise in fear of making the pain worse, or being unsure of what to do and where to start.

5 *Social life*—as with your fitness, you may have noticed that you are going out less and less, and not making plans to meet friends or go on family trips. The uncertainty and unpredictability of your pain may mean that you cannot plan so well now as you are not sure whether you are going to be having a bad or good day.

6 *Work*—you may have had to take time off, you may even have lost your job because the pain became too difficult to manage. You may feel unsure about what your options are for the future and the possibility of working again.

7 *Friendships*—your friendships can be affected as you may feel people do not understand what you are going through, or you may feel that you don't want to 'go on about it any more'. Also, as you may be doing fewer social activities, it can leave you feeling that you have less to contribute. For some people, as their mood drops, they may isolate themselves more and more and as a consequence friendships may change.

8 *Hobbies*—as a knock-on effect of being able to move less or do less, some of your hobbies may become harder to continue. Alongside this your confidence can reduce.

9 *Confidence*—confidence grows as we practice things or continue with things that we currently do. As a response to pain, we often start doing less and confidence can drop. As we become less confident we start avoiding the things that may increase our pain or leave us feeling anxious; however, this in turn leads to us feeling even less confident about doing those very things. It becomes another vicious circle.

10 *Memory*—it is well known that having pain can affect your memory. It is as if your brain is too busy trying to cope with pain rather than helping you focus on and remember things.

11 *Sex*—as your fitness reduces and you start to lose confidence in yourself, your sexual relationships can change. Communicating your needs may be difficult and people often feel uncomfortable talking about sex.

12 *Sport*—as a response to pain you may find that, over time, you reduce the sporting activities you have done in the past. This may start slowly but as time passes you notice that you have stopped all sports. This may lead to feelings of isolation as you stop going out with friends and family.

13 *Finances*—if you are off work or have found that you have had to reduce your hours at work, this will have a direct impact on your income.

14 *Many medical appointments*—this can be because you are keen to find a cure or because you have yet to find any answers to why your pain has persisted. Appointments can lead to further confusion as many healthcare professionals have different opinions.

15 *Thoughts*—it may seem a bit strange to talk about the link between pain and thoughts but, as we will discuss later in Chapter 8, it is quite normal for the things that are happening in our body to influence our thoughts. If your pain is having a detrimental effect on your life you may have noticed that your thoughts have changed. They may be very focused on the pain, they may be focused on what the pain has stopped you from being able to do and they may often be unhelpful. Unhelpful thoughts have a negative effect on our emotions, which in turn can have an unhelpful effect on what we do and how we cope with difficult situations.

16 *Housework*—housework is a form of activity: it is not necessarily enjoyable but something most people want or need to do. As pain builds and fitness drops it can become harder to keep up with normal routines.

17 *Sleep*—many people find their sleep is affected by pain. You may find it hard to get to sleep, you may wake at night and you may find it hard to return to sleep. Also, if you are stiff and find staying in one position difficult then you will wake often during the night. Some people also report that when they try to sleep they start worrying about things and then cannot get off to sleep.

18 *Self-esteem*—it is understandable that when you are not doing the things that are important to you, or that you enjoy, this will have some effect on how you feel about yourself.

19 *Concentration*—as with memory this is known to reduce as a consequence of having pain.

20 *Self-care*—there can be a reduction in, or loss of, your ability to care for yourself and to be independent (e.g. bathing, having a shower). Not being able to do this has a knock-on effect on confidence and mood.

21 *Wearing certain clothes*—for example high heels, tops with buttons, shoes with laces or buckles—becomes difficult, either because they increase your pain or because your fingers do not seem able to manage, or you cannot reach your toes anymore.

22 *Weight gain and body shape changes*—these can change as you are less able to exercise and keep fit.

23 *Doing less*—this happens as a consequence of many of the things mentioned above: if an activity leads to increased pain, it is tempting to then do less of that activity. The next time you have a go, you may worry that it will

lead to another increase in pain. The unhelpful knock-on effect is that as you avoid more, you become more fearful and then more avoidant.

24 *Energy levels*—as a knock-on effect from doing less overall and perhaps having bursts of activity, you can feel more tired, less energized and more lethargic.

25 *Medication*—if taken appropriately, medication can help with some pain. Many people find, however, that over time, medication can become less helpful, the side effects can increase and so they want to stop taking the medication (see Chapter 7).

26 *Control*—as a consequence of all the things mentioned here, many people with pain say that they feel they have no control over their pain and hence their life: pain seems to be taking over.

Many of these things are interrelated. For example, if someone begins to walk less because of their pain, they find that their muscles become weaker and walking becomes harder. Because they find it hard to walk they stop going out with their friends, but because they stop going out they feel more isolated and low in mood. Low mood makes them feel less motivated and so they stop doing the things they enjoy and from which they gain a sense of achievement. Then they begin to think that they cannot do things very well and begin to lose self-confidence, and so on.

Although it can be very easy to recognize many of these things, it can be harder to know what to do and how to make changes to begin to stop them happening and to reduce the effect that the pain is having on your life.

You may have visited many healthcare providers (e.g. doctors, physiotherapists, nurses) who will have tried different ways to help reduce your pain such as injections, surgery, medication or acupuncture. Although they can help some people, unfortunately they don't help everyone—or may only help for a short period of time. Sometimes visiting many people in the hope that they will be able to help you can cause more difficulties because each person may tell you something different and this can be confusing. People often say they feel disappointed after these appointments because they hear that nothing can be done to help them.

Learning pain management strategies will not necessarily cure your pain; this will depend partly on how long you have had it for but also how much your pain has affected your life. However long you have had your pain, pain management strategies can help to reduce the effect it has on your life and help you to improve the areas discussed above. It will take time and motivation to learn these strategies and, more importantly, to use them alongside everything else you do in your life.

Pain management strategies can help you gain control over your pain. It is not easy; if it was, this book would not be needed. In this book we will discuss the strategies that you can start using to enable you to feel more in control of your pain and of your life.

Section 2

Medical treatments

5

What different types of professionals could help?

⊃ Key Points

- There are many different healthcare professionals involved in helping people who have pain and this can be confusing
- Understanding what other healthcare professionals do can help you to understand what they do
- Treatments that you are offered should help you improve what you are able to do yourself as well as help reduce or manage pain

There are many different types of healthcare professionals (HCPs) involved in helping people with pain. Most specialize in one area of treatment or management. To help you make informed choices about your own healthcare, it is important that you know what they do, what they can offer you and what you can expect from them. For those with long-term pain, these HCPs will try to reduce your pain but no one will be able to offer a 100 per cent guarantee of a cure.

It is very important to remember that ongoing pain is not necessarily due to current tissue damage (e.g. of the muscles, ligaments or joints), but rather to changes within your nervous system; your 'hard wiring' (see Chapter 2). Hence, many treatments that focus on correcting your tissues may not give you long-term relief or change what you are able to do. All treatments should aim to improve the amount you can do and your confidence in managing your pain by yourself. It is interesting to know that scientific evidence shows that people manage pain better if they are helped to develop skills to do this themselves. Any hands-on treatment you receive should be part of your treatment time or appointment; the remaining time should be spent teaching you self-management ideas that you can put into practice.

Below we have listed HCPs commonly found within the NHS or private practice who treat people with long-term pain.

Physiotherapist

A physiotherapist is a professional who treats and prevents physical disorders, injury or dysfunction. They prescribe stretching and strengthening exercises and give general fitness advice where appropriate. They also give you information about your condition and how to manage it yourself. Physiotherapists have to be members of the Health Professions Council.

Physiotherapists specialize in varying areas, such as musculoskeletal care, paediatrics (children), neurology (strokes), respiratory (breathing) and oncology (cancer). A small number specialize in the treatment of long-term pain.

Most physiotherapists mainly treat acute pain (short term) and use a number of treatments including manipulation, mobilization, electrical treatments (ultrasound, transcutaneous electrical nerve stimulation [TENS] and others) and exercises. All these are commonly known as 'hands-on' physiotherapy. Some physiotherapists will give acupuncture or administer injections. Those working with people who have long-term pain will not rely solely on using hands-on treatments as there is little evidence to support its use in people with long-term and persistent pain.

All physiotherapists, like other rehabilitative HCPs, will encourage you to do exercises at home or at a gym but the level at which you start is low and progression is gentle (see Chapters 11 and 12).

Nurse

A nurse is trained to care for people who are ill or disabled. Most have special training in the care of patients with particular medical problems. Nurses work in most areas of healthcare and can be one of the first points of contact when you want some healthcare advice. Some nurses also give out TENS machines, are trained in acupuncture and can prescribe some medications and treatments.

Nurses working in pain management departments assist with medical procedures (see Chapter 6), support individuals who would like to review their medications and make suggestions for change. This is done alongside your local doctor or pain specialist. Some specialist nurses can give advice on relaxation and sleep strategies.

Clinical psychologist

A clinical psychologist has a psychology degree and will undertake further specialist qualifications in the care of clinical patients. Psychologists are not medical doctors; they are non-medical specialists who can talk with you and your family about emotional and personal matters. Some help people manage their emotional or psychological responses to injury or disease, and develop ways in which they think and respond to situations.

Psychological intervention involves individual sessions where family members may be able to join work, or working with people in groups.

General practitioner

General practitioners (GPs) are medical doctors who diagnose and treat a wide range of health conditions that can have physical, emotional or social causes. They talk to and examine patients to diagnose their condition and work from community-based premises. They can give patients advice on health issues, prescribe medicine or treatment, perform minor surgery or, where appropriate, refer patients to other healthcare providers. They also educate patients about healthy lifestyles and have responsibility for preventative programmes, such as health screening and influenza vaccinations. For many people, GPs are their first point of contact with healthcare providers. They often act as a central store for medical information like medical notes and letters.

Pain medicine doctor

Pain medicine doctors are specialists who have undergone a basic medical degree. Some have trained in anaesthetics and then gone on to learn how to treat people with long-term pain.

Pain doctors are often the first point of contact for patients who are referred for specialist treatment to a pain clinic. They will have more time than many other medical specialists to take a full history of the problem with an examination as necessary. They are able to perform technical procedures such as spinal injections or give specialist drug advice. Pain consultants almost always work as part of the multiprofessional team so that any one person can get the benefit of many different approaches to help manage long-term pain.

Rheumatologist

A rheumatologist is a doctor who specializes in the treatment of arthritis and other rheumatic diseases or inflammatory disorders affecting joints, muscles, bones, skin and other connective tissues.

Anaesthetist

An anaesthetist is a specialized doctor responsible for your well-being before, during and after surgery or medical procedures. They can administer local and general anaesthetics. As mentioned above, many pain doctors were first trained in anaesthetics and then become pain specialists.

Spinal surgeon

A spinal surgeon is a specialized surgeon who performs surgery to correct problems with the spinal bones (vertebrae), discs, or nerves of the lower back.

Neurosurgeon

Neurosurgeons are specialist doctors who operate on the brain and spinal cord, and other parts of the nervous system.

Orthopaedic surgeon

An orthopaedic surgeon is a medical specialist who performs surgery to bones, joints and ligaments. Orthopaedic surgery corrects problems that arise in the skeleton and its attachments: the ligaments and tendons. They may also deal with some problems of the nervous system, such as those that arise from injury of the spine.

Occupational therapist

An occupational therapist (OT) evaluates the self-care, work and leisure skills of a person. They plan and implement social and interpersonal activities to develop, restore and maintain the person's ability to accomplish activities of daily living (eating, dressing, bathing) and necessary occupational tasks. They help people reach their maximum level of function and independence, to achieve a fulfilled and satisfied state in life. Occupational therapists can provide programmes to help people gain as much independence as possible, for example making meals, carrying out leisure activities or accessing the workplace.

Counsellor

Counsellors help people who want to explore their feelings by offering them time, attention and respect in a private and confidential setting. They usually have a broad training but some specialize in certain areas, for example relationship counselling, bereavement or depression.

Psychiatrist

A psychiatrist is a medical doctor who has specialized in psychiatry and is certified in treating psychological difficulties. They can prescribe medication.

HCPs that give manipulative treatments

There is good evidence that manipulative treatments, performed by qualified clinicians such as physiotherapists, chiropractors or osteopaths in the first 6 to 12 weeks of pain onset can be effective in reducing pain. As with all treatments, if you do not see beneficial changes within three to four appointments, then it is worth reviewing its usefulness. Beyond 6 to 12 weeks after onset of pain, the evidence is that manipulative treatments are less beneficial.

You may find the disciplines below within the NHS, but they are much less common than the mainstream disciplines we have discussed so far.

Chiropractic treatment

Chiropractic treatment involves diagnosing and treating mechanical disorders of the spine and musculoskeletal system with the intention of affecting the nervous system and improving health. Treatment consists of a wide range of manipulative techniques designed to improve function of the joints and muscles. In this context, manipulation means when your joints are moved out of their available range and you hear a click or crack. This is not harmful and is known to cause a short period of relaxation to the surrounding area. The British Chiropractic Association represents over 50 per cent of the chiropractors. Practitioners may be registered with the General Chiropractic Council, the UK's statutory regulator for the profession.

Osteopathy

Osteopathy works towards a balanced and efficient body, by detecting and treating damaged parts. Osteopaths treat a variety of common conditions including changes to posture during pregnancy, babies with colic or sleeplessness, sports injuries and other conditions. The General Osteopathic Council regulates its members and all practising osteopaths should be members.

Alexander Technique

The Alexander Technique is a technique of body re-education and coordination. The technique focuses on the self-perception of movement and its practitioners advise it for alleviating back pain, promoting rehabilitation after accidents, improving breathing, playing musical instruments or singing, amongst other applications.

Acupuncture

Acupuncture is chiefly based on Chinese medicine, attempting to cure illness or relieve pain by inserting needles through the skin, tissues and muscles. In its traditional form, it is thought to help with the flow of energy that is thought to be blocked and restore the body's life energy and balance (called Chi). Fine needles are inserted at specific points along the meridians just under the skin to stimulate, disperse and balance the flow of energy, relieve pain, and treat a variety of long term, acute and degenerative conditions. The Western style of acupuncture stimulates the body through the use of the same steel needles placed in areas where the pain is experienced. The mechanism of acupuncture benefits is not clear but there are a number of studies showing it to be useful in musculoskeletal pain.

Many HCPs are trained to do acupuncture but as with any HCP, you need to know that they have had proper training and are appropriately qualified. You can ask any HCP to tell you about their training and expertise.

Reflexology

This is the practice of stimulating the hands and feet as a form of therapy. It is based on the principle that there are reflexes in the feet, hands and ears that correspond to every part of the body. Reflexology assumes that the entire body is mapped onto these reflex points which associate each organ in the body with a spot on the individual's foot, hand or ears. It is important to recognize that there is little evidence to support reflexology in pain management. That is not to say that some people do not find it helpful.

Summary

This lists the commonest medical disciplines and the treatments which may help in the treatment of pain, but it is not exhaustive. If you are wondering about the benefits of any particular treatment, healthcare providers will often be able to give you advice but they will only be able to work within their experience and training.

6

Can my back pain be cured by injections or surgery?

Written with Mr James Allibone, Consultant Spinal Surgeon, National Hospital for Neurology and Neurosurgery

 Key Points

- It is important for you to make an informed decision about any treatment you plan to receive: the pros, cons and alternatives should all be clear to you
- A balance of different approaches is likely to be more successful than focusing on one aspect; for example, consider lifestyle issues and fitness as well as any one medication or treatment
- If they are right for you, injections or surgery may make you feel well for anything from several months to years. It is important to use this benefit to increase your activity and general health
- Graded increases in movement, stretching and exercise will maximize the benefits of any treatment

Introduction

There are many treatments offered to patients with back pain by way of 'interventions' using injections, implantable devices or surgery. Some of these will be smaller undertakings (such as injections) and others may be much larger where you should anticipate an extended period of recovery (such as surgery). There are also different types of practitioners that might offer things. Interventional techniques depend on the training of the individual providing them and this varies from one practitioner to the next. Table 6.1 is a generalized list of these practitioners and the services they offer.

Table 6.1 Types of specialist

Type of specialist	May offer ...
Rheumatologists or general practitioners	Injections to tender areas or joints reachable without X-ray
Pain specialists, anaesthetists or radiologists (usually offer)	Injections to nerves, spinal joints, discs and bones (often X-ray-guided) and epidurals
Pain specialists (sometimes offer)	Permanent spinal implants
Surgeons (sometimes offer)	Caudal epidurals and other X-ray-guided injections
Surgeons (usually offer)	Spinal surgery with a large variation in the types of operation (see below)

In general terms, wherever you see a lot of variation in practice, this means that there is no clear right answer for which technique is the best practice. It also reflects the range of skills that people attain as they are learning and developing their practice.

You should try to make an informed decision about your treatment as a partnership with the practitioners that you see. A medical consultant is likely to have a broad experience of your problem and will be able to give you advice based on this. You should be given alternative treatment options and the benefits and risks of one choice over another should be fully explained. The options should be tailored to fit your individual need, but will also reflect the skills and experience of the consultant that you see.

The aim of this first part of this chapter is to help you with this decision-making process. The remainder of this chapter describes some spinal conditions and a number of treatments associated with each one. It cannot be stressed strongly enough that every patient is different and that each case needs to be assessed and discussed with a clinician who has appropriate skills and experience.

Some general principles

The best way to approach healthcare is to think of it as being made up of many parts. There are things you can affect yourself and things you may need help with. If you take the example of high blood pressure: a healthy diet, improving the amount of exercise you do and medication will all help to modify your blood pressure and also reduce the risks of a heart attack or stroke.

Your back and musculoskeletal system is another example where activity, exercise, rest, medication, and a positive mental and emotional state helped by support from people around you will all work together to minimize the effects of back pain on your life (see Chapter 2). Focusing on any one aspect of this is likely to mean that another part goes wrong; for example, too much exercise can actually make you have a flare-up of pain, which in turn makes you disheartened and may mean you need extra medication. A balanced approach is the best way and it is accepted that the right balance of things will be different for everyone.

Have a balanced approach to your back pain

- Have a plan to improve your physical condition
- Think about how you might adjust your social and work circumstances to give more focus and time for your condition
- Encourage people around you to support you by explaining what your plans are
- Use drugs where they are helpful
- Discuss the options for treatment with the clinicians looking after you
- When considering interventions, think in particular about:
  - what you are trying to achieve
  - what are the possible adverse effects
  - what is the likely duration of benefit

...and don't be afraid to ask clinicians what the chances of improvement are for any interventions they are suggesting.

Side effects and adverse events are possible after every procedure. People may have unexpected reactions to any part of a process or medicines. It is common to warn people about potential infection, bleeding, failure to achieve the expected effect and worse pain. Serious adverse events are rare after injections (in the region of 1 every 10,000). Complications can, of course, occur after surgery. Your surgeon will explain the type and chance of complications for any operation they recommend.

Making the most of benefit from treatments

Any invasive treatment is best backed up by a graded return to previous levels of fitness and activity. So after recovering from surgery or an injection, gradually increasing what you are able to do will maximize the benefit of the treatment and is the most likely way you will achieve a sustained benefit from it. If you are unsure what you can or should do, then please seek advice. In general, you should not try to achieve too much at once. Start in very small steps, check you can manage and that there is no increase in pain one or two days later, and then carefully stage an increase in activity spread over several weeks. Keeping a diary of what you are able to do can help you to increase in small graded steps.

Spinal injections: epidurals or nerve root injections

Typically, a mixture of local anaesthetic and a locally acting, anti-inflammatory steroid is injected. The effect of the local anaesthetic is temporary, coming on after about 20 minutes and lasting for a few hours. The steroid takes effect over a few days, and may give benefit for days, weeks or months.

There are three common targets for injection:

1 *Nerve root injection.* This places the tip of a needle close to where an individual nerve leaves the spinal column, the so-called 'nerve root'. They are used for diagnostic or treatment purposes in people who have pain radiating from the back down the leg in the distribution of a spinal nerve, for example for sciatica. The injection is often guided using X-rays or a CT scanner.

2 *Epidural injection.* This places the tip of a needle just outside the membrane surrounding the nerves in the lower spine (known as the dura, hence epi-dural, meaning 'around the dura'). They are used for nerve pain and back pain.

3 *Facet and sacroiliac joint injections.* These place the tip of the needle into or around joints in the lower spine. Again, they can have a diagnostic as well as a therapeutic role and are similar in principle to injections in other joints such as the knee or shoulder.

The length of benefit of these injections is variable and unpredictable. Most usefully, they can provide a window of reduced pain during which time you can increase activity and exercise. This may help break the cycle of pain and inactivity, leading to a more permanent reduction in pain. The number of injections will be limited by the total dose of drugs being injected and the amount of X-rays being used.

Evidence for injections

As discussed elsewhere, long-term pain arises for a variety of reasons. Spinal injections may temporarily reduce pain (and this may aid the diagnosis) or they may improve symptoms for many months. Studies in this area have been of variable quality and produced a variety of different results; as with all studies, they generalize for a group of people who have undergone a treatment. Injections for people with pain radiating from the back down the leg may be helped by targeted steroid injections, especially in the short term. The evidence supporting injections for back pain on its own is less compelling. Injections are more effective if performed early on in the development of the condition.

Implants

There are two different types of spinal implants used for people with back pain: spinal cord stimulators and drug infusion pumps.

A *spinal cord stimulator* is used when people have neuropathic pain affecting the lumbar or sacral nerve roots, i.e. pain that is coming from some dysfunction in the nervous system in a pattern relating to the lower limb nerve supply. Using an external controller, the patient uses the stimulator to send small electrical signals to an electrode that lies in the epidural space and stimulates the nerves directly.

An *intrathecal pump* is an implanted pump that delivers pain medication directly to the cerebrospinal fluid (that bathes the spinal cord and nerves) in the lower lumbar region. It needs topping up at regular intervals.

The nature of an implant means that an operation is required to put the device underneath the skin and fat of the abdominal wall. You are usually able to feel it and often there is a slight visible bulge. As the implant is metallic, a variety of alarms will be set off when you walk through them, such as airport metal detectors. Some other electrical systems can also cause interference, for example in libraries or when you go to have certain types of scan (such as MRIs). Modern stimulators and pumps are recharged through the skin but still require occasional battery changes when it wears out.

The commitment to having the device is long term. Although tempting to think that a machine can fix everything, in practice these devices only help a few people and they do not take away all the pain, they simply make it more bearable. They do not change the underlying condition. Many centres require potential patients to have a number of counselling visits before an implant is used.

There are a number of things that can go wrong with implants: they may suffer mechanical failure, the leads may fracture or move out of position, and they have the potential to become infected.

Surgery

People have a tendency to focus on the proposed benefits of surgery. You should also consider how you will feel if the surgery is not successful, or if it leaves you worse off than before. These are definite possibilities. Initial positive results also may not last.

Surgery

Surgery is offered as a solution to specific symptoms. Modern MRI scans reveal many abnormalities in the spine, most of which only need intervention if they are causing symptoms. Surgery offers a predictably high rate of success but this depends on the cases selected. Surgery is much better at dealing with leg pains due to trapped nerves than with back pain itself. Any surgery recommended should be simple and aimed at decompressing trapped nerves. This involves short stays in hospital and is usually considered of low risk. In some cases, particular individual anatomy will require much more complicated surgery, perhaps involving the insertion of titanium screws and rods. This will have a lower success rate and a higher complication rate. In all cases, a recommendation for surgery will be based on a risk–benefit assessment which takes into account factors about the surgery and about the patient. These will be explained to you and should be put in context with the alternatives. If you are not sure you fully understand, then do ask. Feel free to discuss this with your GP, but remember that your GP will have limited experience of all the different types of surgery. Below is a list of different conditions that might be helped by surgery.

Sciatica due to disc prolapse (the slipped disc)

Surgery on disc prolapses may be undertaken if there is MRI evidence of pressure on a nerve from a prolapsed disc and you have associated symptoms. Surgeons hope to operate within six weeks if sciatica is not settling with time or injections. Unless the slipped disc is also causing numbness or weakness, it will be your decision as to whether you wish to be treated with nothing, an injection or surgery. Surgery is relatively minor with a two-night hospital stay. There are some small but definite risks.

Sciatica due to spinal stenosis

Narrowing of the spinal canal can occur with age-related changes in the lower spine. Surgery may be able to improve your symptoms if leg pain or weakness are becoming intrusive, but it may be possible to manage the early stages of the condition with injections. Surgery is usually a little more major than that for disc prolapses, involving three or four nights in hospital.

Back pain on its own

Surgery is sometimes performed for patients with back pain in the absence of leg pain. Such surgery remains controversial. Typically, surgery is relatively major and involves either a fusion or an artificial disc. Careful thought by both the surgeon and the patient is required before proceeding down this route.

Scoliosis

Scolioisis, or a curve in the spine (to the left or right when looking at the back from behind), occasionally needs correction if the curve is getting worse even if there are no other symptoms. More often, the presence of scoliosis is a complicating factor in the choice of treatment options for patients presenting with back or leg pain. Your doctor will explain the relevance to you.

Spondylolisthesis

This is a slip not of a disc but of a vertebra, one of the bony building blocks of the spine. This is not a dangerous condition. In the absence of symptoms it can usually be left alone. It may cause leg and/or back pain. The symptoms are sometimes managed with injections or surgery depending on a number of factors, the most important of which is patient choice.

Summary

Injections and surgery are interventional procedures that may have a role in the care of some people's back pain. It needs to be considered on a case-by-case basis. The best decisions are ones where you and your doctor have had a full and frank discussion where realistic explanations are given for what is being considered. It would be wrong to think that surgery is the answer for most back pain problems: it may be part of a solution, but in the majority of back pain cases it is not the right way forward. Any interventional treatment should be backed up by a graded increase in movement, stretching and exercise in order to maximize the benefits of the treatment.

7

Can I take medications for my pain?

➔ **Key Points**

♦ Medications that can be helpful for pain come from different classes of drug e.g. simple pain killers, antidepressants shown to have a pain-reducing effect, and medications designed for nerve-type pain
♦ Many medications come as tablets or liquids and some are available as patches
♦ You should take medications because they are effective at reducing your pain; doctors or specialist nurses can often help you if you want to reduce your medications
♦ It is not common for people in pain to become addicted to their medications. People who need medications to manage their symptoms usually have no problem reducing their drugs if their problem gets better

Medications can have different names and come in different forms. The names often describe something about what they look like or what they do, for example, pills, tablets, patches, creams or pain killers. This chapter will explain more about the different categories of medicine available and how you can use them to maximum benefit. Quite a few people also want to reduce or stop taking medicines and we will talk about this too. In this chapter, the terms 'medication' or 'medicine' are used interchangeably whereas the term 'drug' normally refers to a chemical compound used as a medicine.

'Medications' or 'medicines' are substances that have been manufactured with careful quality control processes, to produce something with a known therapeutic effect. They have been through rigorous licensing procedures which exist for the safety of the public.

Classes of drug

The easiest way of dividing drugs up is by class. A *class* of drugs is one in which all the members of the group work using a similar mechanism. In general terms, drugs used for back pain fall into the following categories (Table 7.1):

◆ simple pain killers, further subdivided into non-steroidal anti-inflammatory drugs (NSAIDs) and paracetamol

◆ weak opioids (an opioid medicine works on a specific type of cell receptor usually found on nerves)

◆ strong opioids (the best example of this class is morphine)

◆ muscle relaxants and

◆ antidepressants.

A note about medication names

Diclofenac, Voltarol® and Arthrotec® all have the same main drug in them. So why do the same medicines have different names? Drug companies name their medicines as they want to, so they can call and market the same drug by a trade name. However, a medicine will always have a 'proper' pharmaceutical name which must be shown on the packaging and which we use throughout this book.

By convention, pharmaceutical names are written with a small initial letter and trade names start with a capital letter. So Voltarol® and Arthrotec® both contain the medicine diclofenac (where 'diclofenac' is the pharmaceutical name). Arthrotec® is actually a preparation made up of two drugs, diclofenac and misoprostol. Misoprostol is a medicine which protects the stomach lining from some forms of damage.

Lastly, you may see 'M/R' or 'SR' to describe 'modified release' or 'slow release' on some forms of medicine.

Medicines requiring a prescription and those not

There is a lot of overlap between simple pain killers available on prescription and those that are available over-the-counter in pharmacies or supermarkets. In the UK, most pharmaceutical agents are available by prescription even though they may also be on sale on supermarket shelves. It often depends whether you pay for your own prescriptions or not as to where you decide to get simple pain killers like ibuprofen or paracetamol.

Route of administration

Medications can be delivered to the body by a variety of routes. Although many are given by tablet through the mouth, there are many other routes, for example

Table 7.1 Classes of drugs

Class	Description	Examples	Important notes
Paracetamol	Simple painkiller working to reduce pain and fevers	Paracetamol, available without a doctor's prescription	Although generally safe, it can cause severe damage to the liver in overdose
Non-steroidal anti-inflammatory drugs (NSAIDs)	Simple pain killers working to reduce both pain, inflammation and fevers	Ibuprofen, diclofenac, naproxen, mefenamic acid, aspirin and celecoxib. Many available without a doctor's prescription	Common side effects are gastrointestinal pain, indigestion and bleeding (with or without pain). Especially in long-term use, they can also cause kidney damage and have been associated with an increase in heart problems (heart attacks and heart failure)
Weaker opioids	Opioid-based pain killers	Dihydrocodeine, codeine, dextropropoxyphene, tramadol. Largely prescription-only medicines	Although effective, these drugs are not considered as strong or dangerous as the 'strong' opioids. For all in this class, common side effects are nausea, vomiting, itching, constipation, confusion, nightmares, hallucinations, dizziness and sleepiness. Tramadol can precipitate seizures
Stronger opioids	Opioid-based pain killers, subject to stringent laws about who can manufacture, store, supply, prescribe and use these	Morphine, oxycodone, buprenorphine, fentanyl, pethidine, methadone. Prescription-only medicines	The side effects of all opioids are similar although the effects vary between individuals. A serious side effect of opioids is the suppression of breathing. Both dependence and addiction are possible in this group of drugs (see text)
Muscle relaxants	These cause skeletal muscles to relax and can be useful in people with troublesome muscle spasms	Diazepam, tizanidine, and baclofen. Prescription-only medicines	Diazepam is additionally very sedative and can be dangerous in overdose or in people who are not used to it. Diazepam is highly addictive. It is used with caution for people with back pain and usually for a very short time only
Antidepressants	These have a useful action in long-term pain which is separate to their antidepressant action	Amitriptyline, nortriptyline, paroxetine, mirtazapine. Prescription-only medicines	This is a broad class of drugs with many subgroups. There are a number of important medical conditions and drug interactions to be aware of

as liquids to swallow or as an injection. Pain medications are often given by one of the following routes:

- oral, e.g. tablet, capsule or liquid
- rectal, e.g. suppository
- topical or transdermal, e.g. cream or patch.

The drug companies know that people don't usually like taking lots of tablets and there are increasing numbers of patches available. These deliver medicine in one of two ways: either locally to the area where they are placed or by delivery to the bloodstream. It will depend on the design, which will be explained by the doctor prescribing the medicine to you and with the medication's instructions in the packaging. Patches can have advantages over tablets:

- some medicines cannot be given by tablet because they will not work properly (because they are inactivated by the body's digestive system before they can do their job)
- patches can remain active for many days and so you can put them on and forget about taking that medicine for a few days as the patch is doing its job
- a patch may have less side effects than a tablet to produce the same effect.

Which medicines should I be taking?

It might seem like a cheeky answer, but quite simply, you should take the medicines which work. Many people are seen by their GPs or in the pain clinic who have been on certain medicines for ages, even years. They have become used to taking them. They readily admit that they do not think the drugs do any good, but have not considered stopping them because they do not know what they would take instead. This last notion is one that you should consider carefully.

> You should take the medicines that work. Just because there are no alternatives does not mean that you should go on taking a medication that does not work very well.

There are many people who stop taking medicines because they recognize that they are not helping and they usually notice some of the following:

- they are more alert in the day
- their memory is better
- they sleep better
- they are less anxious
- they are more like their 'old' selves
- side effects like constipation are no longer an issue

◆ they feel liberated from taking pills all the time

◆ their pain is no different.

There are some medicines that work very well indeed and these should probably be continued; certainly, stopping them should be considered carefully. The right way to plan the use of medications is with a clear idea of what they are for, why you are taking them, and what the alternatives might be. This can be done with a practice nurse, GP or other clinician who has experience discussing this sort of thing.

How do I try and stop my medication?

You should discuss what you would like to do with your doctor or specialist nurse. You should explain what you would like to achieve by reducing the medication. They may not have done this for someone before but they will know or find out a safe way to proceed. There are some general principles for reducing medications used for pain:

◆ Change one thing at a time or you will not be able to tell which change is responsible for what effect.

◆ Make changes gradually. If you have been on some medications for a long time (like a strong opioid or diazepam), it may take several weeks or months to reduce.

◆ If you have problems with strange feelings you think might be related to a withdrawal syndrome (like feeling unusually uncomfortable, irritable, itchy, nauseous or sweaty) then talk to your doctor or practice nurse. You will probably need to make the reduction slower.

◆ If you find your pain is much worse, then you should reconsider continuing to take the medication you wanted to stop.

Worries about addiction or dependence

Doctors do not tend to use the word addiction when medications are being used for patients who have been prescribed them to treat particular problems. 'Addiction' implies that someone has taken a drug that they were not prescribed and often this is illegal, relating to street drugs. Patients can become dependent on medicines; the degree of the dependence and the nature of the dependence need to be considered very carefully because the medicine may be having a good effect on someone's problem.

Issues around dependence require careful consideration with a doctor. Experience suggests that most patients having long-term medications for pain are not dependent. Dependent people show signs that are clear: they ask for higher and higher doses, they run out of medicines before their prescriptions are due, they go from doctor to doctor asking for the same thing and their day-to-day activities revolve around the drugs they are using.

Why won't my doctor prescribe me the drug I want to try?

Any registered doctor in the UK is able to prescribe any drug that is licensed. A drug is given a license based on its use for particular conditions under certain circumstances, for example duloxetine is a medicine for the pain of diabetic peripheral neuropathy (a disorder of the nerves, or neuralgia, giving pain in the feet). However, doctors are allowed to prescribe any drug that is licensed and so duloxetine is sometimes prescribed for other types of pain caused by damage to nerves.

A doctor will decide to prescribe a medication based on the likely benefit and possible risks of an individual patient's case. They will also be likely to choose drugs they are familiar with. Although there is always a first time, they are not very likely to use a drug they have never used before, especially if they feel it is out of their field of expertise. General practitioners often find that clear advice from an expert, for example a pain consultant, can be useful and supportive in the care of a mutual patient.

The final reason why a doctor may not prescribe something relates to cost controls. Many doctors work within groups with a common approach to prescribing. A medicines committee agrees what is, or is not, acceptable within their group and sets an approved list of drugs much smaller than the list of all available licensed drugs. A general practitioner or a hospital consultant may only be allowed to prescribe from this list of medicines, although there should be methods of appeal or ways to challenge these decisions.

Illegal substances for pain

As the last section of this chapter, it is important to mention illegal substances. This means using substances that are illegal to buy, distribute or possess. Included here are cannabis and strong opioids like morphine bought on the street which might be used to help pain. The biggest clinical worry about the use of these is that their quality and strength is not controlled. One batch may be quite weak, and the next batch so strong that it can kill from an overdose very easily. Equally, there may be poisonous substances that make up the medicines because the suppliers or manufacturers have added chemicals which they do not declare.

It is recognized that both cannabis-derived drugs and morphine are used to treat people with pain. Cannabis medications are available in some countries and not others. Many pain doctors would be interested to know if their patients have found cannabinoids helpful for their pain but would not accept their patients taking other street medications. They may involve the help of the local addiction healthcare services.

8

Thoughts and feelings

➡ Key Points

First things first. Having a chapter about thoughts and feelings in this book does not mean that we are suggesting that you are making up your back pain or that it is somehow in your head. The main reasons that this chapter is needed in a book like this are:

- Psychological factors are involved in the way pain comes into everyone's consciousness and thinking. This is totally normal and how human beings function (see Chapter 2).

- Pain can have a detrimental impact on people's lives and this can affect their mood.

- Persistent pain can be harder to cope with if, for example, you are feeling low in mood, frustrated or angry.

Although it takes time and practice, it is possible to:
- reduce the impact that the pain has on your mood;
- prevent your mood from deteriorating; and
- reduce the chances of your mood stopping you from doing things despite having pain.

The relationship between thoughts and feelings

When we talk about feelings in this book, we are talking about emotions or mood. Feelings tend to be one word, for example:

- Happy
- Sad
- Elated
- Frustrated
- Anxious
- Depressed
- Worried

When people are asked, 'What affects our feelings?', some would say 'How I feel depends on what is happening to me. For example, if I was given a car I'd be elated, but if my car was stolen I'd be very angry and upset.' This shows that the situation we are in has a direct effect on our feelings (see Figure 8.1).

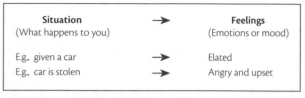

Situation →	**Feelings**
(What happens to you)	(Emotions or mood)
E.g., given a car →	Elated
E.g., car is stolen →	Angry and upset

Figure 8.1 The influence of the situation on our feelings.

It is understandable that people say that feelings are influenced by what is happening to them. However, it is slightly more complicated than this. Take the first example of being given a car. You might think 'It's very kind but I can't afford to run a car. I'm struggling with money as it is but I can't sell it because they will be offended. Anyway, running a car contributes to pollution and I don't want to do that. I don't know what to do.' If you have thoughts like this then you may end up feeling guilty, frustrated and worried.

Take the second example of having your car stolen. You might think, 'Well actually I don't mind. In fact it's quite a good thing. I was thinking of selling my car and getting another but I knew it wouldn't sell very well. This way I can get the insurance money without the hassle of selling it through an advert. At least I didn't lose the car through an accident where someone could have got hurt.' Thinking like this may result in you feeling relieved or even pleased.

These are just examples to make the following important point. It is not just the situation that we are in (for example, having a car stolen) that influences how we feel. It is also the thoughts that we have about what has happened or is happening. Thoughts are very individual to each person. If ten people were in the same situation many of them (if not all) would have different thoughts. This is because our thoughts are influenced by many other things such as our past experiences, memories, health, family circumstances, financial situation and so on.

So the diagram in Figure 8.1 should now look like the diagram in Figure 8.2.

As you can see in Figure 8.2, thoughts can be helpful or unhelpful. The unhelpful ones have a negative impact on feelings (or mood) and can make it harder for us to deal with difficult situations. The helpful ones have a helpful impact on mood and can make it slightly easier to deal with difficult situations. The scientific research into pain currently suggests that certain types of thoughts are particularly unhelpful when someone has pain. One example of this is *catastrophizing*. If someone is catastrophizing they are thinking about the

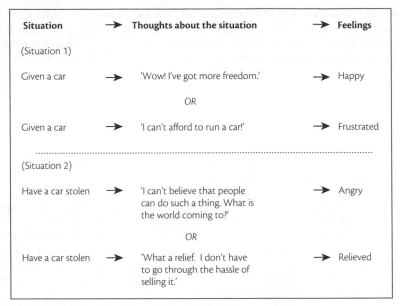

Figure 8.2 Our thoughts about the situation influence our feelings.

worst possible outcomes of an actual or potential situation. People who cata-strophize often think about the pain, its effect on their life and future in a very negative way. There is an association between catastrophizing and:

◆ a higher level of disability
◆ higher levels of depression
◆ low levels of fitness.

An example of this link is described in Figure 8.3.

Other types of unhelpful thinking are listed below in the next box.

Mental filtering

This is when we ignore the positive details and focus on the negative details of a situation.

All-or-nothing thinking

This is when we focus on the extremes of a situation. For example, things are either very good (one extreme) or very bad (the other extreme) or we believe that we have to do things perfectly (one extreme) and if we can't, we don't do them at all (the other extreme).

Overgeneralization

This is when we draw a conclusion that is based on only one single incident or piece of evidence and we then believe that this applies all of the time with everything. For example, one thing goes wrong because of something we did and we end up thinking 'I'm always doing everything wrong.'

Mind reading

This is when we think that we know what someone else will think, feel or act, particularly in relation to us, when we actually don't know.

Fortune telling

This is when we anticipate that things will turn out badly, and we are convinced that our prediction is already an established fact.

Magnifying

We exaggerate the degree or intensity of a problem and make things feel large and overwhelming.

'Shoulds'

'Should' is something we often say to ourselves. For example, 'I should be able to walk further than this.' 'Must', 'have to' and 'ought to' are similar unhelpful words to use. Using these words puts us under a lot of pressure.

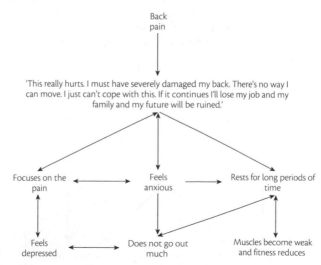

Figure 8.3 The negative effects of catastrophizing.

We all think in some or all of these ways some of the time: it is normal so do not worry if you recognize yourself in many of the above! However, even though they are normal, these ways of thinking tend to be biased and can be unhelpful. For example, they can put us under pressure, make us feel as though everything is going badly or that we are not very good at anything.

The influence of our thoughts and feelings on our behaviour

As you can see in Figure 8.3 about the negative effects of catastrophizing, thoughts and feelings also influence what we do (or our behaviour). Thoughts, feelings and behaviour can also influence what happens in our body, for example our pain (see Figure 8.4).

As outlined in Chapter 4, what we do or do not do can have a helpful or unhelpful impact on our bodies, including pain. A lot of what we do or do not do is influenced by what we believe and think. Hence if we are worried about causing damage to our back, we are less likely to move and exercise. This will mean that our muscles will become weaker, our joints become more stiff and our pain will increase. This might reinforce our belief that our back is damaged (see Figure 8.5).

So what next?

If unhelpful thoughts have an unhelpful impact on the way we feel, what can we do about this? The first thing to consider is that our thoughts are not necessarily fact. Some are, but many are our own interpretation of a situation. Once we recognize this then we are in a position to think about other, more helpful interpretations of the situation. We could do two things. One would be to try and change how we feel and the other would be to try and change how and what we think.

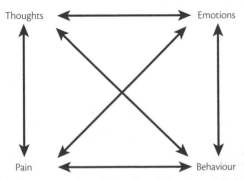

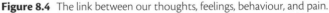

Figure 8.4 The link between our thoughts, feelings, behaviour, and pain.

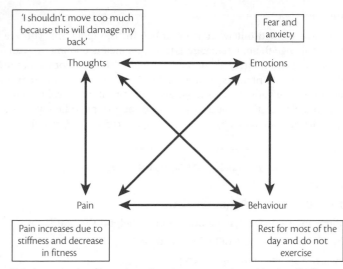

Figure 8.5 An example of how thoughts about your pain and body will affect your mood and what you do.

If we could just 'snap out' of our feelings, chances are we would have done so by now. Changing our feelings directly is very hard; some would say impossible.

Knowing that our thoughts influence how we feel means that we are in a position to do something useful to improve our mood. Replacing one set of thoughts about a situation with a different set of more helpful thoughts will have a beneficial influence on our feelings. Replacing one set of thoughts with another is called *challenging our thoughts*.

Challenging our thoughts takes time, patience and practice. There are several steps to challenging our thoughts.

Step one

First, it is very helpful to become aware of how and what you are thinking and how you are feeling. Because thoughts can be automatic you might first notice how you are feeling. If this is the case, you need to work out what you are saying to yourself to be making you feel like this. It can be helpful to write down your thoughts: they tend to be very fleeting and will go out of your head quickly but leave you with the associated unhelpful feeling.

Step two

Once you have worked out what your unhelpful thoughts are, you are in a position to challenge them. Challenging thoughts means coming up with a different and more helpful interpretation of a situation. It does not mean thinking positively: it means thinking in a more helpful and realistic way. It is important that you believe your challenges otherwise they will not have helpful effect on your mood. You can ask yourself a series of questions to help you begin to challenge unhelpful thoughts. Some of these are listed in the box below.

Questions to ask yourself that will help you to challenge unhelpful thoughts

◆ What is the evidence for my thoughts?

◆ Is there any evidence that supports a more helpful thought?

◆ What other way is there of looking at this?

◆ How can I think about this differently?

◆ Is this way of thinking really helping me at all? If not, what kinds of thoughts would help?

◆ Is my thought fact?

◆ Am I thinking in one of the unhelpful patterns (above) such as all-or-nothing thinking or catastrophizing?

◆ What can I do to check out if my thought is correct?

◆ If my prediction is very likely to happen, what can I do to help me to cope when it does happen?

◆ Can I remember similar situations in the past that will help me to think in an alternative, more helpful way?

◆ Am I asking myself unanswerable questions? e.g. 'Why me?'

Step three

Table 8.1 gives some examples of thought challenges.

Having identified your unhelpful thoughts and challenged them with more helpful thoughts, it can be useful to reflect on whether your feelings have changed. This change may only be small, but even a small change is an important step. It means that you are gaining control over your feelings.

Trying out something to see how realistic your unhelpful thought is often helps changing thoughts and beliefs. For instance, you might be thinking, 'I shouldn't stretch too much because I will suffer from a massive increase in back pain.' You may decide to test how realistic this thought is and stretch for 15 seconds using the principles discussed in Chapter 13 on stretch and movement,

Table 8.1 Thought challenges

Unhelpful thoughts	Emotions	More helpful thought challenges
'My pain is ruining my whole life. I'll never be able to do anything worthwhile again.'	Worry Depressed	'My pain has certainly affected my life but maybe I'm generalizing too much. It hasn't ruined everything. I don't play football anymore but I go to the gym at my own pace and see my friends. I can still go to work even though some days are hard. Some of the things I do even though I've got pain are worthwhile. I help my wife to look after our daughter; the department that I work in is central to the company; and I sometimes forget that seeing my friends and being there for them is certainly worthwhile. I think it'll be helpful if I begin to recognize more often when I'm catastrophizing and generalizing.'
'I find it so hard to believe doctors when they tell me that they can't find anything wrong. Maybe they're keeping something from me or not doing their job properly. My spine must be damaged for me to have so much pain.'	Angry Despondent Worried	'OK, I really have to think about what the physiotherapist told me. She said things heal in about three months and so any pain I have can't be due to damage but that it's more about my pain system and messages. It's safe to exercise. Maybe the doctors are doing their job properly but it's just that it's very hard to find a definite cause for long-term pain.'
'No one seems to understand me or my pain. Why do they think I can keep up with them? Why do they seem to disbelieve me when I say that I can't do something even though I maybe did it the day before?'	Frustrated Resentful	'Maybe I can't expect everyone to understand me and my pain all the time. After all, I don't look as though I'm in pain. I don't use a stick, I don't have my arm in plaster. To most people I look "normal". Constant pain is such a hard thing to understand if you don't suffer from it so maybe I shouldn't expect people to understand. In fact it's probably unrealistic to expect anyone to understand 100%. Rather than getting frustrated I should try and explain my pain to those who are closest to me and just try and get on with managing pain and try not to be too affected by those who I'm not as close to.'

and then see how this affects your pain. You may find that even if your pain increases, it may not be as intense or last for as long as you thought and you might even get some benefit from it. This experience will help you to see that your belief that you should not stretch is not realistic and you may replace your thought with 'Stretching slowly and gradually is helpful for my back.'

Conclusion

We all have helpful and unhelpful thoughts. This is absolutely normal. However, unhelpful thoughts can have a detrimental influence on how we feel, what we do and our body. In addition to all the practical techniques that we have discussed in this book, it will be useful for you to become aware of any unhelpful thoughts and try to challenge these with realistic, more helpful thoughts. This takes time and practice but it is one of the techniques that you can use to reduce the physical and psychological impact of your pain.

9

Communication

➜ **Key Points**

♦ We communicate using verbal and non-verbal methods

♦ Having pain can make clear and effective communication difficult

♦ We can unknowingly give mixed messages about us and our situation. This can be confusing and frustrating for other people

♦ Assertive communication is an important skill for everyone

Communication is used to convey something to other people. It can be:

♦ verbal—when we communicate using our voices and speech, and

♦ non-verbal—when we communicate using our bodies and facial expressions.

Communication is important because it helps us to tell others so many different things such as how we are feeling, what we are thinking, what our needs are, what we would like other people to do to help us, or what we would like to do.

Clear and effective communication

This is very important in many aspects of everyone's life. There are times when communication can be hard for anyone, particularly when they are experiencing pain. Pain can be an obstacle to effective communication in many ways. For example:

♦ pain can make it hard to concentrate on what you want to say;

♦ frustration and other unhelpful emotions that may accompany pain can get in the way of effective and clear communication;

♦ misunderstandings and resentment about pain and its impact can build up between two people which in turn can make communication hard;

♦ the side effects of some pain medication such as dry mouth, foggy head and tiredness can make communication even harder.

Problems that can arise from unclear communication

Difficulties with communication can lead to more problems such as increased pain, tension and anger, which can make communication even harder and so the cycle continues. This can result in some relationships and friendships breaking down. Some of the results of unclear communication are described in more detail below.

Mixed messages

For example, when you are vacuuming, your body language is saying, 'Help me!' Your body is tense, your face has a grimace and you are grunting. Yet when asked if you would like help you shouted 'No, I'm fine!'

Misunderstandings

You are having a bad day and you snap at a friend even though they have not done or said anything wrong. Your friend thinks you are snapping at them and they become resentful, uncommunicative and you both end up in an argument.

Frustration

A big part of you wants to do something without help, so you struggle on and do not ask for help. Your friend becomes frustrated because you look as though you need help but are not asking and your friend knows that if only the two of you did the task together it would be done in no time at all.

Resentment

You are walking with your partner in the park but you begin to find walking harder because your pain is increasing. You think that your partner should know that you will find walking in the park hard and should slow down. Because they are not slowing down and appear not to understand your situation you become very resentful.

People not getting their needs met

You are at work with a group of your colleagues and you all decide to go for a drink after work. One of the confident members of the department says they want to go to a small bar down the road. Although you know that there are very few seats in the bar which is often crowded and you find it hard to move, you do not say anything for fear of making a fuss. You all end up going to the bar, but you have to leave after half an hour because you find it hard to stand any longer.

Things you can do to improve your communication

There are some strategies that you can use that will help you to help your communication become clear and effective.

- ◆ Before you talk to someone, think about and plan the message that you want to get across to the other person.
- ◆ Choose a good time for you to talk (e.g. when you are not tired or when you are not feeling frustrated).

- Choose a good time for the other person to talk (e.g. not as soon as they get in from work or not when they are tired and about to go to bed).
- Choose a good place to talk (e.g. a quiet place where there will not be any interruptions).
- Avoid giving lots of information all at once. Instead, give them small amounts of information at different times.
- Check that the other person has understood what you have said (e.g. 'Just so I know I've been clear, can you tell me what you think I've just asked you').
- Be clear about whether it is a good or bad day in terms of your pain, but tell them this in an assertive way, not passive or aggressive (e.g. 'Just to let you know that I'm having a bad day today').
- Be clear about what you can and cannot do (e.g. 'I can vacuum the lounge and cut the vegetables, but I can't vacuum the rest of the flat, I'll do that next week').
- Be clear about what you would like the other person to do and not to do (e.g. 'Please can you cut up and cook the meat and potatoes and I'll do the vegetables. That's all I'd like you to do, I'm fine with everything else. Shall we aim to eat at 6 o'clock?').
- Remember that the other person has needs and has the right to disagree with you and say no if you ask them to do something.
- Listen to the other person. They also have a point of view and opinion.

What is assertive communication?

Assertiveness can be thought of as being in the middle of a continuum, with passiveness at one end and aggression at the other. Examples of assertiveness are given in the box below.

Examples of assertiveness

- Saying 'yes' when you want to
- Saying 'no' when you want to
- Being confident about handling conflict
- Being able to communicate and negotiate when two or more people want different outcomes
- Being able to give and receive positive and negative feedback

---

Passive behaviour can involve being meek and mild, not telling people what you need or would like. Many of us grow up being told that we should not put our own needs above other peoples or that we should not upset the apple cart. Although this may be helpful to do in some situations, if we do it all the time we very rarely feel listened to, we feel taken advantage of, can feel resentful, frustrated and do not get our needs met. Aggressive behaviour involves putting our rights, needs and wants above those of other people and not considering the latter. It rarely involves giving other people a choice.

Assertive communication helps us to feel better about ourselves, can gain respect from others, helps us achieve goals and reduces the chances of being taken for granted by other people. However, there are downsides to being assertive. It is worth remembering that if you try to decide to be more assertive, it will not always have the desired effect that you want. Some other people may find your assertiveness hard to deal with and respond negatively towards you. They may not like or agree with the views that you are expressing.

How to be assertive

Being assertive is about communicating in a manner that expresses your opinions, rights, needs and feelings in a way that you do not feel taken advantage of, but in a way that also allows others to do the same. It does not involve blaming or judging other people. Here are some things to think about when you are trying to be assertive.

Assertive communication is not just about giving someone your point of view. It is also about *listening to and validating* theirs and showing that you have some understanding of their views. You may find it helpful to start with 'It sounds like you're saying (or you believe). . .'

Assertive communication is about *stating the problem clearly and concisely* and without being apologetic. For example, when visiting a doctor you could say, 'I don't understand why you can't operate on my back when it feels to me that a nerve is trapped.'

An important part of assertive communication is to state clearly *what you would like*. Carrying on from the above example you could say, 'So I'd like you to explain why you can't operate, in a way that I understand.'

In addition to showing some understanding of the other person, stating the problem and stating what you would like, it is important think about *how you say these things*;

Use *'I'* rather than *'you'* as this can feel less blaming for the other person. For example, 'I would like to understand why I have back pain' rather than 'You haven't explained to me why I have back pain.'

Take *ownership* of your feelings. For example, 'I feel angry when you say that' rather than 'You make me angry when you say that.'

When you ask for something, be clear and direct and *avoid being apologetic*. For example, 'Will you please. . .' rather than 'I'm sorry, but would you please' or 'would you mind if. . .'

Sometimes it is important to *keep stating what you want* as the other person may not be listening or may try to change to focus of the conversation. In this circumstance the 'broken record technique' can be helpful. This is clearly stating what you would like over and over again (but still keeping in mind the above points). For example, 'I understand what you're saying but I would like you to . . .' and then if they try and avoid the issue, say again, 'Yes, I fully understand what you're saying but I would like you to. . .'

It is not just what and how you say things but it is also the way you look that affects communication. Non-verbal behaviour is an important aspect of communication. Being passive often involves avoiding eye contact, face lowered down, or looking anywhere but at the person you are talking to. However, too much eye contact can be perceived as aggressive so it is important to get the right balance.

Communication at work

Communicating to work colleagues and managers can be fraught with decisions about whether to say anything to them, what to say to them and when to say anything to them. Although there are no hard and fast rules about talking to people who you work with, it may be worth thinking about the following.

◆ Is your pain getting in the way of you doing your job effectively?

◆ Are you putting all your energy into getting to and from work and doing your job and therefore feel very tired and in more pain when you are not at work, for example in the evenings and at weekends?

◆ When you are at work are you constantly trying to hide your pain and the effect it is having on you?

If you are answering 'yes' to some or all of these questions, then it may be helpful to think about talking to someone at work about your pain and about what you and they can do to help the situation. After all, if you are managing your pain more effectively at work you will probably be more productive.

Some people believe that they cannot talk to their managers about their pain because it would result in them losing their job and not being employable. It is a matter of weighing up the pros and cons of telling your employers. However, they have a legal duty to protect you and to care for your health at work.

If things are becoming unmanageable at work because of your pain and you do decide to talk to your employers, we have listed a few things to consider. Some are discussed above, but some are more specific to the work environment.

◆ Make a list of what you are managing well and what you are struggling with.

◆ Think about the things that you are struggling with and ask yourself what you need from your employer to be able to do them more effectively.

- ◆ Think about whether there is anything that your manager or colleagues could do to help you manage these tasks more effectively.
- ◆ Make list of the main points that you want to get across to the person you are going to talk to. For example:
  - Where my pain is
  - How my pain affects me in relation to my job.
  - What I am managing well at work
  - What I need to be more effective
  - What I need to do differently at work and find out if that's OK by my manager
  - What my manager or colleagues could do to support me with this.
- ◆ Think about the best way to come across to your manager. For example:
  - Get the balance between communicating confidently about what you need to do differently and realizing that your managers need to ensure your work is being done to a good standard and within a reasonable time.
  - Be confident rather than apologetic.
  - Ensure you tell them what you are doing well in addition to what you are struggling with.
  - Tell your managers the advantages to them and your work productivity if they put into place some of the changes that you are suggesting.
  - When you are arranging the meeting find a time that is mutually convenient for you both and do not try to squeeze the meeting into a small time space.
  - Give your manager a clear but brief outline of what it is that you would like to discuss. This could be done verbally but you may be clearer if this is communicated by email or letter.

If you are going to try and change the way in which you communicate remember that assertive communication is a skill and, just like any other skill, it will take time and practice to improve. We cannot always communicate effectively and even if we do it does not mean that the outcome will always be what we want.

Section 3

Self-treatments

➜ Key Points

- Pain can have a detrimental effect across many areas of people's lives
- People with pain can find themselves in many unhelpful cycles, but can find it hard to break these cycles
- When pain has lasted for longer than three months then, because the pain is less likely to be caused by damage, medical treatments may not help the pain. Therefore, learning a self-management approach will be useful
- A self-management approach to pain is about developing skills to help manage pain so that its physical and psychological impact are reduced, and people are able to live a more fulfilling life in spite of their pain

So far we have looked at the back, pain and treatments. Here is a summary of the main learning points from previous chapters.

- Pain that has lasted for longer than three months is not necessarily caused by damage. This means that because there is no damage, there is no healing that needs to take place.
- Medical investigations and treatments may be helpful for back pain. However, if healthcare providers are not offering them it is because they think they will not help your pain.
- Resting for long periods can be more harmful than helpful. It can cause other physical, psychological and social knock-on effects.
- Pain is not mind or body but both. Whenever we experience pain, a mixture of physical and psychological factors are involved.

The rest of the book is about the things that you can do to break out of any unhelpful cycles that you may have found yourself in.

10

Relaxation

➲ Key Points

- Relaxation is useful because it is incompatible with tension and it can help to manage difficult times and situations
- There are many relaxation techniques but the people we have worked with find abdominal breathing, muscle relaxation and body scanning very useful
- Relaxation is a skill that can take time and practice to develop. Try not to be put off if there are some days when you find these techniques hard to use—this is normal

Many people with back pain feel they need to relax. They may feel that their stress levels are increasing or that their muscles feel tense. Relaxation can help in the following ways:

- Engaging in relation techniques means your body is doing something that is incompatible with tension and so it reduces tension.
- Using relaxation techniques during a stressful situation may help you to manage that situation more effectively as they can calm your mind.

As with many pain management techniques, it is important to remember that relaxation is not necessarily about reducing the intensity of pain. It is more about trying to stop unhelpful cycles such as increased tension and stress and to try and prevent the pain from increasing further.

There are numerous relaxation methods. Here we will describe two that, from our experience, are the ones that are easiest to integrate into day-to-day life. You do not have to take yourself away from what you are doing in order to practice these techniques, unlike others where you have to find a quiet room for about 30 minutes, and you do not need any equipment such as a CD player to do these.

Abdominal (or diaphragmatic) breathing

There are times when many of us breathe in our upper chest, allowing the air to only go into the upper half of the lungs. This type of breathing tends to be quite shallow and fast. After a period of time it makes it hard for the body to be relaxed. Abdominal breathing happens when we breathe into the lower half of our lungs. This type of breathing is deeper and slower.

If you wish to try abdominal breathing:

♦ Position yourself as comfortably as you can.

♦ You may wish to close your eyes. If you prefer them to be open, allow them to focus softly on something in front of you.

♦ Become aware of your breath and the movements in your chest and abdomen.

♦ Gently place one hand on your chest and one on your abdomen. Become aware of which hand is moving up and down the most. If the hand on your chest is making more movement then it will be useful to change this pattern and begin to breathe into the lower part, rather than the upper part of your lungs. You may find it more helpful to place both hands on your abdomen with your middle fingers just over your tummy button and their tips touching slightly. If the tips of your fingers do not move apart when you breathe in then you are breathing from your chest rather than your abdomen.

♦ Take a breath in through your nose and gently breathe out through your mouth. Try not to force your breath or breathe deeply, but keep your breath natural. Be aware of your breath moving further down than your chest and into the lower half of your lungs.

♦ When you breathe in your abdomen should rise (and if you have both hands on your abdomen the tips of your middle fingers may part) and when you breathe out your abdomen should fall (and the tips of your fingers come together again).

♦ Ensure that you breathe slowly and comfortably. If you feel able, you can try to make your out-breath slightly longer than your in-breath.

Try to do at least six breaths like this, and more if you have the time.

Muscle relaxation

This relaxation technique is one of the longest. However, we suggest that you practice it as once you are practiced you will be able to do a shortened version.

The technique is as follows:

♦ Position yourself as comfortingly as you can.

♦ Focus on your breath for a short period of time, being aware of your abdomen moving up and down.

♦ Take your attention down to your feet and relax your right foot whilst imagining the tension draining away. You may find imagery helpful. For example, you may imagine a tense foot being blue and then, as you are relaxing it, imagine your foot turning to a warm red. If you prefer not to use colour you can use something else such as texture. You may imagine a tense muscle being hard like a brick and relaxed muscle being soft, like a feather pillow. The use of images is very individual and it may take a while for you to play with different images to see which, if any, you find the most useful.

◆ Take your time and move up to all areas of your body. You can decide how to group the areas but we have made a suggestion in the box below.

Relaxation sequence

Right foot	Lower back
Right leg below knee (back and front)	Upper back
	Right shoulder
Right thigh (back and front)	Left shoulder
Left foot	Neck
Left leg below knee (back and front)	Jaw, cheeks, tongue, eyes, forehead
	Right upper arm
Left thigh (back and front)	Right elbow and lower arm
Buttocks	Right hand and fingers
Pelvis	Left upper arm
Abdomen	Left elbow and lower arm
Chest	Left hand and fingers

Body scan

In this context, a body scan can be thought of as a brief version of the muscle relaxation above. The idea behind a body scan is to scan your body for tension and when you find it, to relax the areas as described above. You can scan all or just some of your body. For example, if you know that you tend to become tense in your shoulders, then you may scan your shoulders at regular intervals throughout the day.

Body scanning is a very useful technique when you are in the middle of an activity or task. It can be as long or as short as you like.

As with many pain management techniques it can be useful to link a technique with an activity that you do regularly every day. For example, you may decide to do a body scan when you are waiting for the kettle to boil or every time you visit the toilet. This means that you do not have to find extra time to do these techniques and they are easy to fit into your day.

Relaxation is a skill that needs to be learnt. Some people will find it harder than others and most people find that some days it is relatively easy to do but on other days it is hard, especially during times of increased pain. It is worth remembering that this is normal and it does not mean that you are someone who cannot relax or that you are doing the technique incorrectly. Give yourself time to practice these techniques and adapt them to your needs. What one person finds helpful, another may find unmanageable. Here are examples of how people have used these techniques.

Examples of when relaxation may be useful

- ◆ Body scan before you get out of bed
- ◆ Abdominal breathing whilst doing the daily stretches
- ◆ Muscle relaxation when you get home from work
- ◆ Body scan whilst standing in a queue
- ◆ Abdominal breathing whilst driving
- ◆ Body scan on your shoulders and low back every 5 minutes whilst working at a computer
- ◆ Muscle relaxation when you wake up at night

Remember

Relaxation is not necessarily about reducing your pain: it is aimed at reducing tension to prevent a further build up of tension and pain. It can help you feel more able to manage the day.

11

What is the role of exercise and movement?

⮕ Key Points

◆ Pain on movement does not always mean that you should not move

◆ Exercise or movement done little and often is better than a long session once a week

◆ You are more likely to continue with exercise if it is fun, something you want to do and done with others

◆ Exercise can help stop pain increasing

◆ Exercise should be social, fun and rewarding

Many people with pain are unsure whether they should exercise or not. It can be hard to know whether to keep going and push into the pain, or stop doing anything that makes the pain worse and rest until it settles. This is confusing and people can find themselves in a cycle of decreasing fitness and increasing pain; on days of less pain it is tempting to do more and on days of more pain it is tempting to do less and rest. However, both of these alternatives can have knock-on effects that can make the pain worse over time.

As well as the many well-known health benefits for your heart, blood pressure and lungs, exercise is an important part of the management of pain, both as a direct treatment for acute pain and as part of the management approach for long-term pain.

The aims of exercise when you are in pain or have lived with pain for many years are to:

◆ help you move more easily, with less stiffness;

◆ reduce the unhelpful effects of inactivity on your body;

◆ increase your general fitness level, endurance and stamina;

◆ increase the amount you can comfortably manage;

♦ help you feel more confident about your body's ability to move; and

♦ help you to be more confident when arranging future activities and making plans.

For some people, exercise may reduce pain. For others it helps keep the pain at a more manageable level.

Part of the aim of this chapter is to find out if the myths about back pain and exercise are true. For example, many of us hear people say to a friend or family member 'come on—no pain, no gain' or the opposite: 'well, don't do if it hurts'. The rest of the chapter will try to answer some key questions that you may have about back pain and exercise, including:

♦ Should I exercise when I am in pain?

♦ Will exercise make my pain worse?

♦ What exercises can I do?

♦ Is there a right and wrong way to exercise?

♦ If it hurts when I exercise, am I doing it wrong?

♦ Can I get back to the sports I used to do?

♦ I have never really enjoyed exercise; do I have to do it and how often?

♦ When do I need to see a physiotherapist or other sports professional?

The myths about pain and exercise

The widely held myths say 'no pain equals no gain' or 'let pain be your guide—listen to your body'. Whilst it is important to listen to your body and understand it, it is essential to know what you are listening for and then what you can do about it.

Should I exercise when I am in pain?

It is very common for people with pain to stop exercising and to avoid movements which can stir up the pain. Exercising may cause you to worry about the added discomfort of aching for hours or days afterwards. It is not surprising then that exercise is avoided. People often think that pain when exercising is a warning sign that damage is occurring and hence stop. For many people this can be very frustrating, particularly if exercise was previously an important part of their lives. However, the opposite to this is also true as pain can get a lot worse and more intense if you keep still and do not move your back. The confusion arises when you go to move the area after resting it and it hurts more.

It would be understandable to think that that pain confirms the idea that you should not move your back or even your legs if it pulls on your back. The answer here lies in the incorrect assumption that the pain means 'stop what you are doing'; what the pain is actually telling you is that you are moving in a way that your body is not used to and that you are stretching muscles, soft tissues and joints more than you have done in the past few days, weeks, or months.

Exercises are not dangerous and cannot damage your joints or muscles if they are done slowly, smoothly, gently and based on what you are currently doing.

A new injury

Samantha has always done a lot of exercise and goes to the gym four times a week; she has developed a sore back with occasional leg pain over the last six weeks. Samantha puts this down to using a new piece of equipment at the gym. She really liked it and used it a lot. She has now stopped using it and can only manage doing a little at the gym.

Muscles and joints in your back like, and need, to be moved. They need movement to maintain their health and vitality, and if they are deprived of this they very quickly tighten up, weaken and get thinner. The way forward is to move your back a little and often. Even by moving it a little you will start to help reduce pain and maintain healthy joints and muscles. You need to find a balance between over-exercising when you have no or little pain and doing nothing when the pain returns. Doing a little, gently and slowly every hour will be better than an hour in one go at the gym. Interestingly, those who exercise little and often (hourly or daily), get fitter and looser much faster than those who do big bursts of exercise once a week.

Will exercise make my pain worse?

Many people with back pain will have already experienced their pain increasing after doing something physical, for example mowing the lawn, swimming or going to the gym. Doing too much, and the way you exercise, can make some exercises aggravate your pain. This is normal. Healthy, fit people also feel aches and pains if they try to exercise after a period of inactivity or do something which they are not used to. This is training pain; it is not harmful and cannot be completely avoided, although it can be greatly reduced by increasing exercise and activity gradually, just as athletes do in their training. As you get fitter these aches and pains associated with training will reduce. Some people enjoy this feeling as it tells them they are working the right muscles, but if you already have pain, you do not want any extra, especially if it will result in you doing less the next day.

Experiences like this after exercise may make continuing with exercise difficult. For example if exercises (or other activities) are overdone, then increases in pain are likely. If the levels of increased pain become too much, it may lead people to think that it is not worth continuing to exercise—or that it is harmful. Flare-ups or increase in pain lasting 2–48 hours, are often a result of trying too hard, perhaps when trying to prove to others or themselves that there is no gain without pain, or even when pain levels feel low and the temptation to do a bit extra can be very strong. In the past you may have exercised a lot, pushed hard and found this training pain a sign that you had done well. However, pushing muscles that already hurt will not reduce pain but instead increase it with spasm and soreness.

If specific exercises do make you more sore and the pain lasts into the next day, then rather than stop the exercise altogether see if you can reduce the range, intensity, or weight. Remember, this pain is probably telling you that you are working muscles and joints that are weak and stiff and hence it hurts. The exercises need to be done more often but with less range or repetition—little and often.

What exercises can I do?

It is important to recognize that people prefer different types or ways of exercising, for example because they find them more enjoyable, or they can exercise with friends or family members.

It is not the type of exercise you do that is the key but the way you go about it.

The key is to introduce exercise slowly, at a pace that you feel comfortable with and with your least feared movement/exercise first. What helps most with maintaining exercise is the feeling that you are in control of what you are doing and that you feel confident with why you are doing it the way you are.

> Exercise needs to be a way of helping you increase not just your fitness but, more importantly, your confidence in doing things: the amount you do day to day, for example, to reach for top shelves, carry more shopping or sit on the floor. Activity-orientated exercises are more important than exercises that focus purely on range of movement. It should not be seen as a chore, but rather as a means to an end—to be able to do more fulfilling things in life.

It can be helpful to ask yourself when you last did any exercises and what they were. If you have not done them in the last few weeks then you need to start even lower than you think and then, as your body gets used to them, build up.

Stretch

Stretch is the area of exercise that can be most underestimated in the management of both acute and long-term pain. Stretch, if done slowly and gently, is very good for our bodies. Our muscles benefit from it, our ligaments benefit from it, as do our nerves. It keeps the tissues flexible and supple, brings the circulation into the tissues and the lubricating fluid to our joints. When you are warmed up, an exercise can have a bounce to it, but for stretching it is best to go slowly and hold the stretch steady, without bouncing.

The soft tissues in your body are like elastic bands, if you stretch and release an elastic band quickly it will simply return to the original length without lengthening, and the body behaves in much the same way. Take the stretch only to the point of first resistance, and not increased pain. A good way to monitor this is to observe your breathing. If you push the stretch too far you will probably find that it affects your breathing pattern and you may even hold your breath. You can breathe as a way of timing the stretch. One normal relaxed breathing cycle (in and out) is about 3 to 6 seconds, depending on how you breathe. When you stretch you should aim to hold the stretch steady as you count 5 to 10 normal breaths.

It may be helpful to gradually build up the amount of time you hold the stretch for. For example, if you find it too difficult to hold for five breaths then you could start initially holding for one breathing cycle and gradually build up over days or weeks. The important point, though, is to be consistent with the amount of time you stretch for and not change the count from day to day depending on your pain, that is not allowing your pain to guide you.

Don't repeat stretches in quick succession; it is likely to place your muscles into cramp or spasm—this can be really painful. Sustain stretches and repeat strengthening exercises, building up repetitions as you get fitter and more used to them.

See Chapter 13 more information on stretches.

Is there a right and wrong way to exercise?

As we have said, the key to exercising and fitness is to do things slowly, gently and smoothly but also that you build up your exercise and fitness levels in a systematic, planned way. This is pacing—a systematic, incremental approach to building on the amount of an activity and exercise that can be easily managed.

Pacing is a means to an end, a strategy that can allow you to increase your fitness and exposure to everyday activities in a gradual way. It will help you gain more confidence and control over your fitness, as it moves you from a pain-dependent approach to a more helpful, time-dependent approach.

An old, recurring injury with long-term pain

Martin has had back pain on and off for 15 months, but has complained of a stiff back for many years. He recently did lots of DIY at home and has since had more pain. He is generally fit and active but does very little exercise above his day-to-day activities and work.

Like many people with longer-lasting, long-term pain, Martin was finding it hard to know what the best thing to do was. He did not know whether to keep going and push into the pain, or stop doing anything that made it worse and rest until it settles. Martin found this very confusing as he knew that both of these alternatives could have knock-on effects that can make the pain worse over time. Martin could already see, though, that he was starting to avoid doing more than he had to and had stopped nearly all DIY. He had found himself in a cycle of decreasing fitness and increasing pain; on days of less pain he was tempted to do more and on days of more pain do less and rest.

If it hurts am I doing it wrong or is it supposed to hurt?

To gain anything from stretch there should be a feeling of stretch, but not be an increase in pain. Think of stretching to a borderline—if the part you are stretching has pain in it at the time, stretch until you begin to feel an increase in resistance, or tightness and then stop there, between your pain and more pain. If you do not feel pain in the part you are stretching all the time, stretch until you begin to feel resistance coming on, not pain, stop there, at the borderline between no pain and tightness. Try not to push into the pain: this will increase muscle pain and tension, and will minimize the benefit of any stretch you will have achieved.

Remember that a strong stretch is like a mild burning feeling. Sometimes when you first stretch a painful joint it hurts, this is actually very much like the burning feeling of a strong stretch. If you start gently and slowly, the joint will become suppler and in time you will find you can move further before the feeling of stretch starts—the borderlines change. A lot of people believe that the harder you push and force a joint the looser it will become. This could not be further from the truth—in fact you will only set yourself back and cause your muscles to go into spasm and consequently cause more pain. Soft tissues in our bodies respond best to slow, gentle and smooth movements.

There are three signs you can look out for which might indicate that you are pushing the stretches too far. If you feel yourself doing these when you are stretching then take a few deep breaths and start again in a gentler way:

1 holding your breath, grunting or groaning

2 clenching your fists or tensing your shoulder muscles

3 screwing up your face and gritting your teeth.

Another sign of stretching too much is when you feel the muscle aches or is more sore for more than two hours after you have stretched. If this is the case it does not mean that you should stop doing the stretch; rather, the next time you try to stretch, do not push the stretch as far and ensure that you are able to keep breathing normally. You could also reduce the time (the number of breaths) that you hold for as well.

Can I return to the sports I used to do?

The key thing to understand is that there is no rush with increasing exercise and activity levels and that it is the slow, gradual approach that enables long-term change and produces the best outcome. This approach will also build your confidence to challenge avoided, difficult and feared activities and movements.

The key to becoming more active is to not push exercises, but use muscles in a relaxed way. Then build up *gently* and *gradually*.

We would encourage you to do whatever exercise or sport you like. Some may be more advanced than others, in that in order to do them you need to be very fit, but there is no reason why someone with back pain should not go horse riding, swimming, or running. If you wanted to go on a hack for four hours but hadn't been on a horse for a year then the goal is too big, but if you wanted to sit on a horse for five minutes and had been building up your inner leg strength and hip flexibility then that is an appropriate way to start, and you can build up gradually.

I have never really enjoyed exercise; do I have to do it and how often?

Exercise, in that it leads to increased activity levels, is of course important for more general reasons, such as returning to social activities, improving general health (aerobic fitness for cardiac health, weight-bearing exercise for bone strength, and so on), and the overall benefit of being able to join in with friends and families in such normal things as going for walks, bike rides and going on holidays.

If exercise is not your favourite pastime, it needs to be seen as a means to an end. If by exercising you are able to walk further or play football with your children then the 10–15 minutes you take out each day to do the exercises may be well worth it.

The kinds of exercise that ideally would be included into your exercise routine are:

◆ *Stretching.* To help stiff and tight joints, muscles and scar tissue to loosen up and become supple again. Stiffness adds to discomfort, altered posture and restricts daily activities. For best results stretch should be done *gently, slowly* and *daily.*

◆ *Strengthening.* To build up weak and deconditioned muscles, so that they can support joints and help you do more. This is best done three to four times a week, unless your day-to-day activities are similar.

- *Aerobic*. Building up the stamina of heart and lungs (being less out of breath upon exercise or activity). This has many other benefits:
  - reduces blood pressure
  - improves muscle tone and endurance
  - improves sleep
  - improves weight control, along with a healthy diet
  - gives an improved feeling of well-being (endorphin release).

Aerobic (cardiovascular) exercise increases your heart rate to a target range that is set according to your age. Your heart rate should be kept within this range for 15 to 20 minutes each time you exercise and this should be done three to five times a week. Initially you will only able to exercise to your tolerance but as you continue your ability to exercise for longer periods will increase.

When do I need to see a physiotherapist or other sports professional?

It can be helpful to review the way exercises are done with your physiotherapist. For example, are they slow, smooth and gentle? Do you need more advice on relaxation and incorporating appropriate breathing with exercise, or more information about pain and your body? The physiotherapist should be consistently encouraging about exercise, giving advice like 'do it gently within *your* manageable range and you will not damage yourself' is often very useful. The physiotherapist can provide reassurance that training pain is likely, and that a stiff joint may feel rusty when stretched. This information and reassurance can help you to keep going when starting to exercise. Physiotherapists expect some reactions and difficulties, know they are normal and know that there will be an end benefit.

I have been told I have scar tissue—what should I do?

As mentioned in Chapter 1, scar tissue is created by the body during all injuries. It is actually a very helpful and vital substance but not if it becomes tight and pulls on surrounding tissues. Scar tissue adapts well with stretching and its natural properties to tighten can be greatly reduced. Again, the key is slow and gentle stretching.

12

How much activity can I do?

> **⊙ Key Points**
>
> ◆ It is important to be consistent in the activity you do
> ◆ Try not to do more on a day where you feel less pain and less on a day where you feel more pain
> ◆ Timing how long you do things for and sticking to these times can help

Setting goals and having targets of things to work towards is important

As a result of long-term pain many people change the way they do things. But, as time goes by, one can begin to feel that it is impossible to do anything to change. On better days when the pain is at a tolerable level, it is tempting to do jobs or exercise that were put off when the pain was bad. On days when the pain is worse than the day before, it is tempting to do less and rest more. This is a common pattern of activity for long-term pain sufferers. Good days are a time of particular confusion, because it is easy to do more, resulting in a flare-up in pain later that day or the next. People often rest during a flare-up, but this can result in weaker muscles and a drop in fitness. A vicious cycle thus develops between getting things done and managing the pain.

Although the pain from overactivity subsides, rest makes movement stiffer and painful. This can lead to feelings of frustration at not being able to get things done and even despair, wondering if you are ever going to get on top of your pain. This cycle of activity is known as the (over)activity and underactivity cycle where pain intensity can change. During each period of increased pain it becomes more tempting to avoid certain activities, which you associate with more pain. It is known that pain, when chronic or long term, is not a useful message as it frequently tells us to stop too late or too soon.

Pain can often get in the way of people doing things. This can result in many feelings including disappointment, anger and frustration. If we do not achieve things then we do not gain a sense of achievement or satisfaction; we are less likely to try the activity again and more likely to feel a sense of failure. This is why goals can be important for everyone. Goals (or aims) give us something to work towards, to focus on, to motivate us and to help us gain a sense of achievement in life.

To set your activity goals you need to know how much of each activity you can comfortably manage—we will call this 'baseline setting'.

> *Baselines* are determined by what you feel is manageable in time or amount, when done in a relaxed way and you can also manage on your worst days. Your baseline is always within your present capabilities.

A baseline is the point from which exercises and activities can begin. It is also the amount of activity which is easily manageable (measured in time or number of repetitions), which can be done comfortably, and does not cause a flare-up in your pain (that is pain levels increasing above normal for a period of more than two hours after the activity). Pain which remains high within two hours but for no longer is due to the stretch or exercise being new and can be often be talked about in terms of 'rust' from that movement.

Baselines need to be established over several days (ideally two or three and at different times), to allow for any natural fluctuation in day-to-day pain levels. Measurements can be made using time or a number of repetitions. The baseline is determined by taking the average of those measures achieved over the trial days and reducing this by 20 per cent. Thus the baseline is 80 per cent of the average. From this point you can decide on the pacing *increments* for each stretch or exercise and activity. When you start a new exercise, movement or action, there is likely to be some training pain. A sensibly low baseline and a slowly increased pace will help keep training pain to a manageable level and in the long run lead to a much better outcome.

Pacing

The aim of pacing is to help you to find a way to start new activities or previously avoided activities. It may provide you with new ways to do things without causing an increase in pain later. As stated earlier, pacing is a way to do more but yet not increase your pain levels further. Pacing helps you plan and carry out activities in a way which gives you more control and allows you to plan your future by breaking activities down into small, manageable parts.

Pacing is a process of building up from your baselines so that you can do more and more of your chosen activity, hobby or exercise. Once you have decided how you are going to build up your activity—i.e., the increment—it is important and key that you stick to them, good day or bad. Remember that your body will be the same from day to day, your muscles will not suddenly be looser and stronger and hence cannot manage big changes in the amount you ask them to do.

This is the hardest part; not being tempted to overdo it on a good day, or miss out your activity when the pain feels worse.

Often people need to reduce the amount they are doing on their good days as they are doing too much. This activity can then be built up again more slowly alongside stretches. This can often feel like a backward step but it is not—initially you will slow down but long term you will be able to do more without paying for it later. Baseline setting and pacing are essential in order for fitness to be built up and are increased weekly or daily so that they do not cause increases in pain which usually lead to a reduction in activity.

Once you have become accustomed to regular exercise/activity, you can gradually increase it to improve fitness levels. It is a good idea to set a limit so that you do not try to do too much too quickly, that is, pacing! Some people like to increase by a percentage, for example 10 per cent whereas others like to use a set time, such as one minute.

By using the above principles of baseline setting and pacing, activities you have avoided or are unsure about can be considered. Below are more tips about goal-setting and how to link that to baseline setting and pacing.

Goal-setting

The best way to set goals is to choose an activity or task that you want to improve on or return to and use this as your goal. It may take some time to work out a goal that you would like to work on. There are examples of people's goals in the box below.

Examples of goals

Walk further

Play football with my son

Vacuum the living room without my pain increasing

Return to part-time work

Walk to the park

Get in and out of the bath independently

Feel more confident with bending forwards

Return to the gym

Do not forget that these are examples and may not be what you want to do. Goals are very individual. It is important that your goals are enjoyable or you want to achieve them. There is no point in setting goals that you do not want to do.

It is important to set **SMART** goals. The **S, M, A, R** and **T** stand for particular words.

SMART

Specific: Goals need to be specific so that you are clear about exactly what it is that you want to achieve.

Measurable: You need to have some form of measurement in your goal so that you know when you have achieved it. Measurement can be many things, including time or distance, such as for 10 minutes, for half a mile.

Achievable: Goals need to be achievable in terms of finance, demands on your time, etc. otherwise you are less to likely reach the end point.

Relevant: It is essential that goals are relevant to you and your lifestyle. There is little point in your setting a goal that you do not feel is relevant for you.

Time frame: You need to put a time frame on your goal so that you know when you want to have achieved it, for example, in one week or in three months time. This will help you to keep aiming for the end point rather than letting things drag on and on, which may result in decreased motivation.

'Be able to walk further' is not a SMART goal. Even though you may think it is achievable you do not know:

◆ how far you will walk

◆ where you will walk to

◆ when you hope to have achieved this by.

Turning this into a SMART goal will make it look something like this:

'In four months time I would like to be able to pace my walk to the local park which is 100 yards from my house. When I get to the park I will sit on the bench, read my newspaper for 10 minutes, and then walk back to my house.'

Specific: Walk to the park, sit down and read paper and walk back home

Measurable: The park is 100 yards away, then I'll read for 10 minutes and then I'll walk the 100 yards back home.

Achievable: Yes, it's achievable and I feel confident I can do it

Relevant: Yes, I always enjoyed reading the paper in the park

Timed: I aim to achieve this goal in four months time

We often think that there needs to be an 'F' somewhere in SMART because it is important that you are *flexible* in your approach to goals. Life can be unpredictable for anyone and things can get in the way of you achieving a goal in the time that you had hoped to. Being flexible about this will help you to change the time frame and not give yourself a hard time for doing this.

When you have decided on your goal, write down all the steps that are needed to be able to achieve this goal. You need to think quite broadly about this. For example, for a goal of going swimming it is not just 'swimming' that you need to be able to do. You need to be able to pack a bag, carry the bag, travel to the pool, get changed, get into the pool, swim, get out of the pool, have a shower, get dried, get dressed, travel back home.

'In four months time I would like to be able to pace my walk to the local park which is 100 yards from my house. When I get to the park I will sit on the bench, read my newspaper for 10 minutes, and then walk back to my house.'

Look at the example above of walking to the park. The components of this goal are:

1   Get up and get dressed
2   Get down the ten steps from my flat
3   Walk for 100 yards
4   Carry the newspaper
5   Sit down comfortably for 10 minutes
6   Hold the newspaper whilst reading it for 10 minutes
7   Walk 100 yards back to the flat
8   Climb the ten stairs to the flat

When you have listed the components, list what it is that you currently find difficult and that is getting in the way of achieving your goal. The person who has set the goal above might write down the list below.

At the moment:

My pain increases after walking about 50 yards

I can only sit comfortably for six minutes before my pain increases

I think I can only hold a newspaper whilst reading it for five minutes

After doing all that I think I'll find it hard to climb up ten stairs to my flat

The key is in being aware of what you feel less or more confident with and starting with what you feel more confident with.

This list gives you an idea of what it is that you need to work on if you are going to achieve your goal. So, for example, this person needs to work on:

Increasing the strength in my legs so that I can increase the distance I can walk

Increasing the length of time that I can sit for

Increasing the strength in my shoulders and arms so that I can hold a newspaper

Increasing the number of stairs that I can climb up

Increasing my general level of fitness so that I can achieve the above

13

Specific stretches and exercises

 Key Points

- There is no right or wrong stretch—it is the way you stretch that is important
- Breathe in before you start your stretch and then breathe out as you stretch
- Build up your range of movement (your flexibility) before you increase your strength/muscle power
- Tight stretches indicate areas that could be causing your pain or impacting upon it; proceed with them as little and often as feels manageable—do not avoid them
- Slowly, gently and smoothly—sustain a stretch. Don't repeat them in quick succession

Warm-ups

Warm-up exercises are just what they say—to warm up your muscles and joints in preparation for more stretches, exercise or activity. Warm-up exercises do not take long, and can be squeezed into any free minute. They can be done at any time and anywhere, and can be especially useful if you have been still in one position for a while, for example sitting in a car, in a queue or in the cinema.

Below are some warm-up stretches which you can try, do each one for a couple of seconds. Remember to do them slowly and gently.

While standing

1 Place your arms by your side, gently turn your body from side to side, letting your arms follow your body and swing round from side to side.

2 Roll your shoulders forwards and backwards, repeat a couple of times each way. As if you are sticking your chest out and taking your shoulder blades together.

3 Gently shake your arms and then each leg.

4 Stand with your feet slightly apart and then transfer you weight from side to side. This can be built up into walking on the spot and then slow jogging and so on building up to running if you want.

Stretches

These stretches can be done all in one go or they can be spread out through the day: the key is to do little and often every day. You can repeat some later during the day if some are more useful and helpful than others, but otherwise do them once. The stretches which are the hardest to do often mean that they are the ones you need to persevere with: the key is to move slowly and smoothly and not to expect quick changes.

Start each stretch by holding it at a *comfortable* level for a count of five seconds. You can build this count up each week or whenever it feels manageable. **Don't repeat each one five times**—this is likely to make the muscle tighter rather than looser.

While standing

1 Take a deep breath in as you stand with your arms by your side. As you breathe out, slowly bend forwards, sliding your hands down the front of your legs towards the floor – the aim is not to reach the floor but go to a comfortable position, be that the top of your thighs, knees or the floor.

2 Place the palms of your hands in the small of your back, slightly lower than your waist. Place your hands so your fingertips are pointing towards the floor and your thumbs out to the side. Then gently arch backwards, as if you are arching over your hands. This is a small movement, and whilst doing the stretch try not to bend your knees. Again, breathe out as you stretch backwards.

3 Take a deep breath in as you stand with your arms by your side. As you breathe out, slowly slide your right hand down the outside of your right leg, so you are tilting to the right. Go only as far as is comfortable and hold for a count of five seconds. Take another breath in and as you breathe out slide your left hand down the outside of your left leg.

4 Bend your right knee so your foot is sticking out behind you and rest your toes and front of your foot on a stool or seat of a chair behind you. Take a breath in and as you breathe out slowly bend your left knee. You may feel a stretch in the front of your right thigh (see Figure 13.1). Repeat with your left leg. Start with a low enough surface so the stretch is comfortable and if you do not have a chair or step near by you can try to use your trouser leg and lift towards your bottom.

Sitting

1 Sitting towards the front of a chair, take a deep breath in and as you breathe out slowly bend forward from your waist and bend towards the floor,

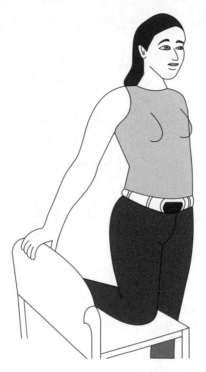

Figure 13.1 Thigh stretch.

go to the point where you start to feel a stretch or your comfortable limit (see Figure 13.2).

2 Take a deep breath in as you place your right hand on your left knee and as you breathe out slowly, turn to look over your left shoulder. The stretch can be as small or as big as you feel comfortable with. As you are able to move more you can turn more from your waist and the stretch will be greater. You can increase the stretch by placing your right hand behind the chair.

3 Take a deep breath in and cross your right ankle over your left shin or knee, whichever is more comfortable. As you breathe out slowly let the bent knee drop out to the side, only to the point of stretch. You can place your hand on your bent knee if you want more stretch. Repeat with your other leg (see Figure 13.3).

4 Take a breath in and as you breathe out gently take your chin downwards to your chest. Return to your starting position, then take a breath in and as you breathe out take your chin up towards the ceiling. Do not repeat this but hold it for a count of five.

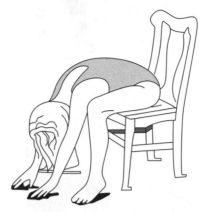

Figure 13.2 Forward sitting stretch.

5 Take a breath in and gently pull your chin in, backwards as if you are making a double chin. Try not to tip your head up or down or move your shoulders forward. This appears to be a small stretch and it is supposed to be. Do not be tempted to repeat it, hold the stretch for a count of five.

6 Take a breath in and as you breathe out gently straighten your right knee out in front of you and pull your toes up towards your knee. You may feel a

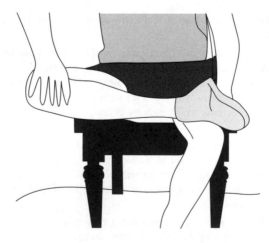

Figure 13.3 Crossed knee stretch.

stretch in the back of your right leg. Hold for a count of five and repeat with your left leg.

While lying

1 Lie on the floor or your bed, bend your knees and rest your feet on the floor and place your arms out to your side. Take a breath in, breathe out and with your knees together roll them from side to side. Only go as far as feels comfortable. The aim is not for your knees to reach the floor. Repeat this five times each way.

2 Take a deep breath in and as you breathe out bend your right knee up towards your chest and if you can easily reach hold your knee with your hands (see Figure 13.4). Don't stretch further if your other leg is coming off the floor. Repeat with bending your left knee up.

3 Take a deep breath in and cross your right foot over your left leg/knee—wherever it feels most comfortable. As you breathe out use your left hand to guide your right knee/thigh/leg across your body to the point of slight stretch. Hold to a comfortable point for a count of five.

4 Lying on your tummy, place your hands level to your shoulders at shoulder width apart. If this feels uncomfortable move your hands upwards away from you shoulders. As you breathe out gently push down through your hands and lift your shoulders and head upwards. Your pelvis stays on the floor/mat/bed.

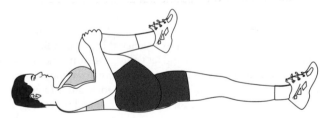

Figure 13.4 Single leg stretch.

Strengthening

There are many ways to build up muscle strength. The best way to keep fit is through your day-to-day activities and general exercise, for example housework, gardening, DIY, cycling, swimming or walking. Many people go to specific exercise classes, like yoga, Pilates or aerobics.

Exercise classes and going to the gym are really good ways of exercising and keeping fit but the same approach is relevant here as it is with stretching. The key is to build up slowly and be consistent in the amount and the frequency of when you exercise. You are more likely to get fitter if you exercise for a shorter period of time but regularly as opposed to once a week for two hours.

If you are more sore after you have exercised it does not necessarily mean you have done some damage: it is much more likely that you have done more than your current level of fitness. You have asked too much of your body that day. The key thing is to start with doing one or two of each of the exercises and each week build them up, being systematic in your increases. Some people may think that this is not worth it but by starting low, you can ensure that you will be there at the end, won't pay for it the next day and then have to miss going because you are in so much pain.

There are also specific exercises that you can do. Below are a few common exercises that physiotherapists give out. Build up the number of times you repeat them. Remember to be consistent in the amount you do, that is do the same each day and systematically increase time and/or repetitions.

While lying

◆ Lie on your back with your knees bent and hip width apart with feet flat on the floor. Tighten your tummy muscles; it is as if you are squeezing your tummy button down towards the floor. The hollow in your back may flatten as you do this and the front of your pelvis may rise upwards. Hold for a count of five and repeat. This is called a pelvic tilt.

You can advance this by then lifting your bottom of the floor so your knees align with your pelvis: this is called a bridge.

On all fours

◆ Kneel on all fours. You may need to practice this position first if your knees need to get used to it. Breathe in and let your tummy muscles relax and hang down towards the floor, as you breathe out gently draw your tummy muscles up. Try not to do this with all your effort, go to about 60 per cent of what you feel you can manage. Hold for a count of five and repeat.

You can advance this by lifting one arm out in front and holding it for a count of five, then repeating and then changing arms.

The best way to keep fit is to integrate exercise into a routine, make it part of you daily life and, if you can, do it with other people. You are more likely to keep it going if you are doing something you enjoy.

Also remember that there is no clear evidence saying that one type of exercise is better than another, rather that you enjoy exercise and your confidence to do it increases and grows.

Section 4

Bringing things together and real patients' stories

The impact of back pain

When people experience back pain for a significant period of time it can begin to have a wide-ranging effect on them, their lives and also on the people around them. People with back pain often say that over the past few months or years they have experienced some or all (and more) of the following:

- Reduction in fitness
- Weak muscles
- Stiff joints
- Get out of breath more quickly
- Stop going out with friends and family
- Lose contact with friends
- Become more isolated
- Do not enjoy life as much
- Changes in work
- Find it harder to manage their work
- Reduce their working hours
- Stop working
- Sleep:
    - Find it hard to get to sleep
    - Wake up during the night

- • Feeling tired throughout the day
- • Sleep during the day, but then unable to sleep at night
- ◆ Medication:
  - • Try many different medications
  - • Take more and more medication
  - • Experience side effects of medication
  - • Medication does not help their pain or only takes the edge off their pain
- ◆ Visit to many healthcare providers
- ◆ Have been told different things by different people about the cause of their pain
- ◆ Have been offered a variety of treatments; some of which may have helped but some have not helped
- ◆ Confusion about what is causing their pain
- ◆ Not knowing what is the best thing to do for them and their pain
- ◆ Feeling depressed, fed up or low in mood. This may be because of:
  - • Feeling unable to achieve anything
  - • Experiencing many losses, for example, job, friends, leisure activities
  - • Feeling hopeless about their situation
- ◆ Anxious or worried. This may be about:
  - • The effect of their pain on their future
  - • Doing certain activities in case it causes more damage and/or pain
  - • Feeling unable to cope during times of increased pain
- ◆ Guilty about:
  - • Feeling unable to fulfil their role as, for example, a parent, a partner, a colleague, the 'breadwinner'
- ◆ Frustration about the pain interfering with many aspects of their life, such as achieving tasks and activities or concentrating.

These are just some of the effects that back pain can have on some people's lives. You may be experiencing just a few of these or many more. Pain can have consequences on many areas of life and it can feel as though the pain is taking control of many areas of your life.

About 40 to 50 years ago researchers and healthcare providers began to recognize that medical treatments do not help everyone with pain. They began to look for another way to help people whose pain could not be cured. The focus was on reducing the unhelpful effects of the pain on people's lives. The techniques have been developed and have become known as 'pain management' or 'self-management of pain'. As these phrases suggest, these techniques are about managing, not curing pain and the person who takes the control is not the doctor, physiotherapist or other health-care provider, but the person with the pain—you. Pain management techniques can be useful at many stages; when pain begins; throughout the time that the person is trying medical treatments; and when all medical treatments have finished.

The aims of self-management techniques are to:

◆ Reduce the detrimental physical and psychological impact of pain

◆ Improve physical and psychological function despite pain

Self-management techniques are described throughout this book and are listed below:

◆ Goal-setting

◆ Activity

◆ Exercise and stretch

◆ Pacing

◆ Thoughts and feelings

◆ Relationships and communication

◆ Medication

◆ Sleep

One of the most important things about self-management is that it is the *combination* of the techniques that will help you to manage your pain. It will be much harder to manage your pain if you just focus on one technique.

14

Coping with a new pain: what can I expect from treatments?

> ## ➡ Key Points
>
> - It can be confusing and worrying when a new pain starts. During this time it can be helpful if you understand chronic pain and know that some pains that seem to be new can actually be part of your long-standing pain condition
> - Using the pain management techniques that are described in this book can help you to manage the pain
> - If the new pain does not settle after a few days it may be helpful to see a doctor
> - If you are offered another treatment is it important that you make an informed choice about whether or not you agree to the treatment

> ## 📄 Case study
>
> Miss Havent (aged 37) has had low back pain for over twenty years. She has seen many doctors over this time. These have included a surgeon, a rheumatologist and a pain management consultant. No one has ever found a definite cause and at least two doctors have given her different diagnoses. She has had many interventions, including injections, physiotherapy, and acupuncture. Some interventions have helped and some have not. None have helped for a long period of time. Four weeks ago Miss Havent noticed a new pain that is a little higher up her back than her usual pain and it feels sharper. At first she thought it was just part of her normal pain and decided to rest a bit more, but it is not getting better and she is now worried that it is caused by something new. Her GP also seems concerned and referred her to a rheumatologist. The rheumatologist said that a course of injections might help. Miss Havent is keen to have the injections but she wonders how much they will help.

'I have a new pain'

People may become concerned if they start to feel a different pain that may be in the same or a different area to their usual pain. Whilst this concern is understandable, it can also be unhelpful. Excessive concern and worry can have an unhelpful impact because it can prevent people from keeping calm and deciding on the best way forward. Understanding pain can help to keep you calm. Chapter 2 explained how pain can start and continue. When pain has lasted for a few months or more, it can spread to other areas of the body. For example, someone who has long-term upper back pain may start to feel pain in their shoulders and neck or low back pain may start to spread to the upper back. The way that the pain feels can also change. For example people often describe experiencing a range of sensations and feelings such as sharp pain, numbness, pins and needles, or an ache. Experiencing a new pain does not always happen but if you have noticed that you are getting pain in new areas it can be helpful to know that this can be normal and, whilst it is unpleasant for you, it does not necessarily mean that your new pain is caused by a worrying new problem.

It is important to think about whether this new pain is or is not related to your usual back pain. If you have overdone an activity, then it may be linked to your usual pain. If you have done a new activity then you may have overdone it. If the new pain does not settle after a few days then you may want to get it checked out by your doctor.

To help you manage this potentially worrying time, it will be helpful to take time to think about your thoughts about the situation. As described in Chapter 8, the way we think influences how we feel and how we cope with situations. If you are concerned about a new pain, it will help you to deal with this and decide on an appropriate course of action if you are able to reduce your worry. As we saw in Chapter 8, this will involve becoming aware of your concerns and what you are thinking and then challenging these thoughts with alternative, more helpful ones that will then reduce your worry and concern. See the box below for an example.

Challenging thoughts about a new pain

When people experience a new pain, they may have unhelpful thoughts such as these:

'I'm really worried about what's causing this pain. I'm sure there's something new wrong. This is the last thing I need. Things will just get worse and worse. I'm struggling already. What will I be like in a few years time?'

Worrying about a new pain is understandable but not helpful. If it is not related to your usual back pain then you need to be calm enough to get the most appropriate help. If it is related to your usual back pain, then keeping calm will certainly help you to think about and put into practice helpful strategies to help you manage the situation.

An example of a challenge to the above thought could be something like this:

'OK, I'm not sure what's causing this pain. It could be something new but it could be related to my back pain. Maybe I'll go to my GP and ask what he thinks. If he thinks I should see someone else, then at least that's a positive step forward. If he thinks it's related to my back pain, then at least I know it's not caused by something new and horrible and I can spend a bit of time thinking about what I can do to help me manage this pain.'

What if a doctor has offered a treatment for the new pain?

You may feel that you need to go and see someone such as your general practitioner, another type of doctor or a physiotherapist when you have a new pain. If you do this, it will be helpful to talk to them about whether they think your new pain is linked to your back pain or whether they think it is caused by something new and whether an investigation and/or treatment may help. If you do have an investigation, remember what has been explained in Chapter 3 and that the results of investigations are not necessarily linked to the pain people experience. So when the results come back, it may be helpful to talk to your doctor or physiotherapist about their meaning. If you do not understand what they are telling you, you have the right to ask them to explain in a way that you understand. Not understanding what is being said to you can be a cause of confusion, frustration and worry.

You may find that you are offered another treatment, such as an injection or hands-on physiotherapy (see Chapter 5). When any treatment is offered, it is important that you make what is called an *informed choice* about the treatment. It is the responsibility of the healthcare provider to provide information that will help you to make the informed choice about whether you decide to refuse or agree to have the treatment. It is important that you think about the things in the box below.

Things to consider when making an informed choice

Investigations:

◆ Why does the healthcare provider think that the investigation may help?

◆ What is involved in the investigation?

◆ If the results show something, what could be the likely treatment?

◆ Is there a chance that whatever the results show, there won't be any treatment?

Treatments:

◆ Why does the healthcare provider think that the treatment may help?

◆ What are the other treatment alternatives?

◆ What is involved in the treatment?

◆ What does the research evidence say about the percentage of people whose symptoms:

• Improve after the treatment;

• Remain the same after treatment;

• Become worse after the treatment.

◆ What are the side effects of this treatment?

◆ When will I start to feel the benefits?

◆ What is the chance that the treatment will cure the pain?

◆ If the pain goes away or reduces after the treatment will this last forever or will it be short term?

In summary, having a new pain can be worrying. However, when someone has long-term pain many new pains tend to be linked to the existing pain. It will be helpful if you are able to challenge any unhelpful thoughts about this situation because this will help to reduce your worry and to make a decision about what to do. The self-management techniques that are described in this book will be helpful for new pains, but if they persist for a few days and you are still concerned then visit your doctor. If you are offered a new treatment then it is important that you make an informed choice about whether to have this treatment.

15

Making sense of scan results and finding a cure

➲ Key Points

- Hearing that nothing can be found to be causing your pain can be very confusing and frustrating
- It can be very tempting to visit many healthcare providers to try and find someone to tell you exactly what is wrong
- However, in the case of long-term pain it is not as simple as this and visiting many people can actually be unhelpful
- It can also be tempting to respond to pain by reducing your level of activity and resting. Again, in the case of long-term pain this can be unhelpful

📄 Case study

Mr Webb is 56 years old. His back pain began for no apparent reason three years ago. He has seen a rheumatologist, spinal surgeon, neurologist, and pain management consultant. They have all sent him for investigations, such as blood tests, X-rays, and MRI scans but all the reports were normal and he has been told that nothing can be found that is causing his pain. Mr Webb thinks that people think that the pain is all in his mind. He has seen the results of his MRI scan and he is sure that the discs in his back are damaged and causing his pain. He desperately wants a doctor to find the cause of his pain because he believes that this will lead to a cure. Not only is Mr Webb worried about what is causing his pain but he is concerned that he is doing less and less activity even though he tries really hard to keep moving on the 'good' days. He believes that if his pain is not cured he will end up in a wheelchair.

Why do people keep telling me they can't find anything wrong?

In many Western cultures we tend to grow up with the belief and understanding that if we have pain then something in our body must be damaged. If people have this belief then they understandably think that if they rest then the damage will heal and the pain will go. However, as described in Chapter 2, when pain persists for longer than about three months this type of pain (called chronic pain, long-term pain or persistent pain) is not necessarily caused by damage. This means that scans and X-rays can appear normal: the person is told that the doctors cannot find anything wrong and yet they are experiencing severe pain. This does not mean that the pain is made up or in their mind, but it does mean that medical science has not yet developed an investigation that can easily show up the exact cause or presence of long-term pain.

It is important that people who have had pain for longer than three months begin to understand their pain in another way other than their pain being caused by damage. Chapter 2 will help you to do this. It means that there is not anything such as a broken bone, or damaged muscle or torn ligament or something worrying, such as a tumour, that is causing your pain. Chapter 3 explains how the results of investigations can come back as 'normal' despite someone experiencing pain. If the results of investigations are normal then this probably means that your pain is caused by the changes in the way that your body sends pain messages as described in Chapter 2.

> When people tell you that they cannot find anything wrong or cannot find anything that is causing your pain, it is important to remember that this does not mean that you do not have real pain.

I'm going to keep searching for a cure

After being told by one doctor that they cannot find anything to be causing their pain, many people ask to see a second, and then a third doctor and so on. Unfortunately this can cause unhelpful knock on effects. Just like Mr Webb, people who have back pain may see many types of doctors and other healthcare providers and have many investigations only to be told again that 'nothing can be found to be causing your pain'. Just being told that 'nothing can be found that is causing your pain' or that 'you do not have any damage' rarely helps to reduce people's concerns about the cause of their pain. Many people continue to think that something must be wrong but it is just that the investigation or doctor did not find the cause. Just as in the example of Mr Webb, this can have three knock on effects:

♦ People continue to feel worried or anxious about the cause of their pain (see Chapters 4 and 8) and so focus on the pain, the effect it is having on their life and seek another healthcare provider who they hope will provide an answer.

◆ They think that other people think that the pain is in their mind or are making the pain up. This can make some people doubt themselves and the reality of their pain which can be very distressing. Other people become very angry and disillusioned with the healthcare system and feel hopeless about ever receiving the right care.

◆ They want to continue their search for someone who will tell them exactly what is causing their pain in the hope that this will lead to a cure. People who have long-term pain often say that they have visited many healthcare providers, all of whom have given them a different reason for their pain. This can be very confusing and can make it even harder to think about what might be the best way forward. Some scan results can add to this confusion. People who are experiencing a lot of pain may have normal scan results and people who are feeling little or no pain may have very abnormal scan results (see Chapter 3).

These knock on effects can have many other unhelpful knock on effects and can lead to a downward spiral. If you have been told by more than one doctor or heath care provider that they cannot find anything wrong with your back to be causing your pain it may be helpful to use this as a signal to yourself to begin to find ways other than seeing lots of doctors to help your situation. This can include the pain management strategies that are listed at the beginning of Section 4 and described throughout this book.

I think that my back must be damaged therefore I'll do less activity

As in the case of Mr Webb, people who are concerned about their pain and the cause of their pain often find that because of their worries and concerns about making things worse they begin to do less and their overall activity level gradually decreases. However, as their level of activity decreases, so too does their fitness. A decreased level of fitness means that their activity reduces even further, and so on (see Chapter 12 for a detailed explanation). When in this situation people can become concerned about what might happen to them in the future if this continues and have frightening thoughts such as 'I might end up in a wheelchair'.

When people's level of activity and fitness decline they often find themselves in the over/under activity cycle, as described in Chapter 12. Just like Mr Webb they have days when their pain has increased and days when it is back to its normal level. People often let their level of pain determine to amount of activity they do. On the days when the pain is at its normal level people tend to push themselves to do tasks because they say their pain will increase later in the day (or week) and prevent them from doing things. During the times when their pain increases they rest. When this pattern occurs for a long period of time people's overall level of activity decreases as does their strength and fitness. This can cause people to worry about the future. However, although it can be difficult to begin with, this cycle can be stopped by using 'pacing' and people can gradually increase their level of activity, fitness and enjoyment of life despite having pain. See Chapter 12 for a detailed description about how to pace activities. The main things to remember when trying to get out of this cycle are:

♦ Having pain does not mean you have damage to your back.

♦ Try to avoid your pain being the guide to how much activity you do. Be guided by time.

♦ Try to do the same amount of activity on a good day and a bad day. Do not push yourself too much on a good day and try to do some gentle activity on a bad day.

As with many if the pain management strategies that are discussed in this book, it is important to be aware of the thoughts and feelings that you are experiencing when you are putting these strategies into practice. For example, when people are learning how to pace their activity they often have unhelpful thoughts such as:

♦ 'I can't pace. It'll slow me down and I'll never get anything done!'

♦ 'Pacing takes all the spontaneity out of my life.'

♦ 'How on earth can I keep moving when my pain increases.'

Thoughts such as these can lead to people feeling:

♦ Frustrated

♦ Angry

♦ Despondent

If you are having thoughts such as these they will get in the way of you pacing your activity and from experiencing another, possibly more helpful way of doing your day to day activity. Although thoughts such as these are totally understandable, they are not helpful. It is therefore important that you try to challenge these thoughts as described in Chapter 8. Possible challenges to the unhelpful thoughts above include:

'Although it may feel as though pacing slows me down, it'll hopefully mean that my pain won't increase and also I'll have less bad days. This will mean I will be able to do something every day of the week rather than just three days and so over the week I may get just as much done, or even more, and hopefully my pain won't increase.'

'Pacing does reduce some of the spontaneity. But I have to remember the reason why I'm learning to pace. It will

mean that eventually I will be able to do more things. As
I become more used to pacing it may feel less restricting.'

'Because my type of pain isn't a helpful signal and it isn't telling me
that my back's damaged then it's safe to move. It may be harder to
move on the bad days but if I take it gently and move in a relaxed
way with short rests in between then I'll be able to maintain a level
of movement that will prevent my body from stiffening up.'

In summary, being told that nothing can be found to be causing back pain is
common, although frustrating, with this type of pain. If you are not sure exactly
what the person who is telling you this means then it is important that you ask
more questions so that you do understand. Understanding your pain will lessen
the chances of you seeing more and more healthcare providers and being told
many things that can be conflicting and confusing. When you have had back
pain for more than three months and people cannot find an exact cause, then
the self management techniques described in this book will be helpful. Although
they will not provide you with a cure, they will help to reduce the psychological
and physical impact that the pain is having on your life.

16

Home life is difficult

→ **Key Points**

♦ Pain can change what people can and cannot do. It can be hard to adapt to this. It will take time and ways to reach this point will be different for everyone. However, there are two things that may help you. The first is about acceptance and the second is about gaining a sense of achievement.

♦ As with many changes that happen in life, having pain can affect your beliefs about and your ability to fulfil the roles that you have in life, for example a wife, son, daughter, colleague, father and so on. Addressing your beliefs and what you can do to fulfil these roles in other ways may help you.

♦ Many people with back pain say that it affects their sex life in physical and emotional ways. Addressing things such as self-confidence, expectations about sex, communication and becoming used to touch can help you and your partner to feel more satisfied about your sex life.

📄 **Case study**

Mrs Patton is 41. She has been married for 15 years and has three children aged nine, six and four. Her husband works full time in a demanding job and Mrs Patton is the person who carries out most of the household tasks and childcare. She has had back pain for three years.

Prior to her back pain Mrs Patton used to be very active, took pride in her house and loved caring for her children. She and her husband enjoyed an active sex life and had sex two or three times a week. However, since her pain began she has gradually enjoyed life less and less. She finds the housework a chore and although she loves her children she finds caring for them hard work. Towards the middle of the day Mrs Patton's back pain has increased to an almost unbearable level.

Mr and Mrs Patton now have sex about once every two months. She finds that sex increases her back pain and Mr Patton has said that he's worried about increasing his wife's pain. Mrs Patton goes to bed before her husband hoping that she'll be asleep before he comes to bed and so they won't have to have sex. Because of all these difficulties Mrs Patton is embarrassed about the state of her house and feels as though she is letting her family down and that her children are suffering. She loves her husband but feels a failure as a wife and she thinks that he will leave her if the situation continues.

'But I used to be so active!'

As we have discussed a few times in this book, when people have pain their level of activity can reduce. This can be hard for many people to come to terms with, especially for those who used to have a high level of activity, such as a busy job, doing all the housework and childcare or being very active with sports. If this is you, there is no quick and easy way to resolve the disappointment, frustration and anger that you may be feeling about this. However, there are two areas that may be worth thinking about. The first is about acceptance and the second is about gaining a sense of achievement.

Acceptance

People often loathe the idea of accepting their pain and the effect it is having on their lives. This may be because 'acceptance' can have many meanings for people. By talking about acceptance we do not mean:

◆ Giving up all hope in the face of pain
◆ Letting the pain take over your life
◆ Realizing that you will never do certain activities again
◆ Embracing your pain with a constant smile on your face

When we talk about acceptance we mean:

◆ Recognizing that you will experience a certain level of pain
◆ Doing meaningful and/or enjoyable activities despite experiencing some pain
◆ Recognizing that your pain will change some aspects of your life but that you can still be in control
◆ Working towards your future in a way that takes account of your pain but not letting the pain being in control
◆ Working with, rather than fighting against your pain both physically and emotionally.

You may find that reading this initially makes you feel angry or low. Try to recognize the thoughts that you are having that influence the way you are feeling.

You may be thinking, 'I can't work with my pain! I just want it to go', or, 'Well, they obviously don't have pain, they've no idea what it's like having pain every day. How on earth can I accept that I have pain every day?' These thoughts are totally understandable. Acceptance (for want of a better word):

◆ Does not happen overnight. It takes time.

◆ Is not a position that you will reach and then stay there. It is an ongoing process that changes in both directions throughout people's lives.

◆ Does not have a specific formula that everyone can apply to themselves. People with pain are individual and will begin to accept their pain and situation in a number of different ways.

Gaining a sense of achievement

As you may be experiencing, pain can get in the way of doing things and therefore from gaining a sense of satisfaction and achievement. People also describe how it can become harder to fulfil their roles in life such as being a partner, a work colleague or a parent. Because they believe they are not fulfilling these roles effectively they lose a sense of achievement and satisfaction and become very frustrated.

There is no getting away from the fact that pain may stop you from achieving everything that you had planned. However, it certainly does not have to stop you from doing many things although you may have to think differently about how you might achieve them. For example, it may take longer to reach your goal now that you have pain; you may need to have more help to reach the goal than you would have previously; or you may have to change the way in which you go about achieving the goal.

When you are thinking about how to gain a sense of achievement, an important must be thing to remember is that your plans and goals must be *realistic* (see Chapter 12 about how to set goals). It may be tempting to plan and set the same goals as you would have done before you had pain. However, this may lead to you pushing yourself in an attempt to reach your goal, which may result in an increase in pain. If you set your goal too high and are unable to reach it, you may see yourself as having failed and feel disappointed and/or frustrated. People often view taking their pain into account when planning goals as 'lowering' their expectations and they fight against doing this. There is not a right or wrong answer to this, but viewing this as lowering your expectations is unhelpful. A more helpful way to look at this may be to see it as changing, not lowering, expectations.

An example may help. Even if it takes a day longer to reach a goal, the fact that you have done so despite your pain is a great achievement and, arguably, an even bigger achievement given that you have pain. People may say 'Yes, but I want to be able to live like I did before I had the pain.' This is understandable. However, not taking the pain into account can result in more difficulties, such as increased pain, increased tiredness, and a feeling of not having achieved anything. When you set goals it is important that you take your pain and your current situation into account.

Some people with pain focus on things that they believe they have failed at rather than thinking about what they have achieved. This is often because they feel that they 'should' have achieved more. This can leave them feeling like a failure, as though they never achieve anything and as though the pain has taken over their life. To help you take into account what you have achieved, it can be helpful to write down your goals, no matter how small you think they are, and tick them off when you have completed them.

Fulfilling our roles: being a 'good' parent, partner, friend and so on

We all have roles in our lives. These may include being partner, mother, son, colleague, daughter, husband, wife, friend and so on. Juggling these roles and looking after ourselves can be hard in today's society. We can feel a lot of pressure to do well at work, be a caring partner, be a great parent, be a supportive friend ... the list can go on. When back pain is added into the equation it can be harder to fulfil these roles to the level that we feel we should be able to and people with pain often talk about not being good enough or failing in these roles. In addition, people with pain can be caught up in the struggle to find pain relief and the time spent focusing on other important aspects of their life diminishes.

Many, if not all of us, have values that relate to areas of our lives such as family, intimate relationships, friends, work, health and learning. For example, someone may want to play football with their son like they used to before having pain but is struggling to do this and constantly feels knocked back and a failure as a parent. Rather than thinking about what you used to do that helped you to recognize that you were a good parent, it can be helpful to think about the underlying values behind what you used to do rather than what you actually used to do. The value behind the example of playing football with their son might be to be involved in activities that bring them and their child pleasure. This will help them think about activities to be involved in other than football or will help them to plan how they might play football with their child despite their pain.

In the above tale, Mrs Patton describes herself as taking pride in her house. However, she feels unable to keep her house as clean and tidy as she once did. Again, it might be useful to think about the value behind the activity of cleaning the house. If she decides that it actually is not that important to her when compared with other areas of her life and that it does not provide her with a sense of satisfaction, achievement or enjoyment then she might decide to focus on activities in her life that do this and plan how she can keep the house in a 'good enough' state. However, she might still feel as though it is very important to her to keep that house clean and tidy and therefore she needs to be able to think about how to do the housework in spite of the pain. This would be helped by using the pain management strategies discussed in this book (for example, pacing, stretching to increase her confidence and flexibility, communicating with her family to help her with the housework, challenging her unhelpful thoughts that may be saying that she is not doing things well enough).

Relationships and sex

Although people tend not to mention it, it is common for back pain to affect people's sex lives. People describe the following problems:

* Sexual activity increases their pain
* They are frightened of and avoid sex because they worry about an increase in pain
* Their partner is frightened of increasing their back pain and so they also avoid sex
* The person with pain feels less attractive
* The person with pain or their partner loses self-confidence and believes that they are unable to satisfy their partner anymore
* The person with pain feels guilty about not having sex so they force themselves to do so but do not gain any satisfaction from sex
* Communicating about sex can be hard due to embarrassment, worries about hurting the other person's feelings or worries about increasing the pain if sex becomes more frequent
* Medication can reduce people's desire to have sex (their 'libido')

On a practical level, stretches can improve your flexibility and also increase your confidence and reduce fear about moving and being in different positions. Stretching after sex can help to reduce stiffness and subsequent increases in pain.

People who have persistent pain can become sensitive to touch so that even the most gentle of touches can feel painful. This can make the person with pain and their partner feel hesitant and worried about touch. There are three things that would be helpful to address here. The first is people's concerns about what the pain means, the second is people's apprehension about touch and the third is about people's sensitivity. All three are linked but for the purposes of this chapter we will talk about them separately.

1 First it is important to understand what any pain and increase in pain means. It will be helpful to remember that increased sensitivity, which is common in long-term pain, can make light touch feel painful. However, this is not related to damage. Touching, stroking, massage or rubbing will not cause damage or harm.

2 Second, when people are apprehensive even before being touched they will be focusing on the possibility of increased pain and therefore will find it harder to focus on pleasure and enjoyment. This will increase worry and apprehension (see Chapter 8 about the effect that our thoughts have on our feelings and what we do). Knowing that you will not cause damage or harm may decrease your worry. It may also be helpful to use short relation techniques during sex to help you relax (see Chapter 10) and feel more focused on pleasure rather than pain.

3 Third, although it takes time, it may be possible to reduce a certain amount of sensitivity. This can be done in graded steps. For example, if someone feels very sensitive around one buttock and the top of their thigh they might gradually increase the pressure they use to touch that area using the steps in the box below.

Example of how to become more comfortable with touch

1 When you are on own and feeling relaxed, gently stroke a scarf across the sensitive area.

2 When you are used to the above stage, do the same but with something that has increased pressure, such as a sponge or a light touch with your hand.

3 When you are used to above stage, increase the pressure again.

4 When you have achieved stage 3, ask your partner to gently touch and stroke you in the sensitive area.

5 For this stage, ask your partner to increase the pressure.

And so on . . .

People's expectations and beliefs can often be a barrier to a fulfilling sex life. It may be helpful to think about the expectations and beliefs that you or your partner have. Some examples of these are listed in the box below. Think about what your expectations and beliefs are.

Examples of common expectations and beliefs about sex

◆ We must have sex as often as we used to
◆ We must have sex twice a week
◆ We must always have intercourse
◆ My partner no longer finds me attractive since I've had pain

---

◆ I'm never able to satisfy my partner

◆ My partner is very unhappy with our sex life

◆ Sex should last a certain length of time (e.g., 50 minutes or at least an hour)

◆ I'm no good at sex anymore

◆ Sex must always be spontaneous

Of course, we are all different, but take some time to think about the expectations and beliefs that you have and whether these are helpful and realistic. Sex can be a taboo subject that does not get discussed and so people do not know what 'the norm' is or may believe that what we see on television, films, or in advertising is the norm. This is a very high and unrealistic expectation for most people to have.

It is important to remember that even when neither partner has pain the frequency with which they have sex changes throughout their relationship. Placing pressure on yourself to have sex as often as you used to may not be realistic, even if you do not have pain.

Pain can affect people's sexuality and they may feel less attractive than they used to. Chapter 8 will help you to think about how your thoughts about yourself affect your sex life. If you are telling yourself you are no good at sex; that your partner is not attracted to you any more; that you will never have a fulfilling sexual relationship; it will have an adverse affect on you and your sex life. It can sound like a bit of a cliché but if you take some time to feel good about yourself then this will have a beneficial effect on your self-esteem. What makes us feel good differs greatly but it may be that a trip to the hairdressers, putting on make-up, buying yourself a shirt, or eating healthily may help.

The demands of modern life can result in sex being put at the bottom of the list for a lot of couples. Add this to pain and tiredness and sex can become even less appealing. If you decide that you do want to improve your sex life then it important to make time to have sex and think about what you and your partner can do together to help you both have a fulfilling sex life. Communication is something that is very important. Try to avoid presuming that you know what your partner thinks and wants. Read chapter 9 on effective communication. Unfortunately people can feel embarrassed and avoid talking about sex. However, a lack of effective communication can lead to many assumptions, and unrealistic expectations. It can be helpful to communicate the points in the box below.

Things that you may want to communicate about

- What you do and do not enjoy
- What you would like your partner to do
- What you would like your partner to avoid because it increases your pain
- What you will be doing to help make sex easier and less painful for you
- What your partner can do to help make the situation easier and enjoyable for you

REMEMBER: communication is a two-way thing. It is important that you listen to your partner and ask them to tell you what they enjoy, do not enjoy, would like you to do, would like you to avoid, and what you can do to help them.

Your partner's beliefs and expectations

It may be helpful to find out what your partner thinks and feels about your sex life. People with pain can get into a cycle of feeling guilty, frustrated, and angry towards their partner. They sometimes say things like:

- they don't understand how painful it is to have sex
- I feel so guilty because I know he wants to have sex more than we do
- I know that he's not happy with our sex life.

Actually, these may be just the beliefs of the person with pain and their partner may be thinking something very different—it would be helpful to find out. If you avoid physical contact your partner may interpret this as you rejecting them (which you may not be). Your partner may be terrified of hurting you and so is frightened of touching you (but you interpret this as them not caring about you). Your partner may remember a time when you suffered from a massive increase in pain after you had sex and so they are assuming that you do not want to have sex (but actually you might be desperate to find a way together to have a fulfilling sex life).

If you have read this chapter and identify with some of the issues that we have raised, then it may help to know that many people with pain experience difficulties in their sex lives. Many of the difficulties that arise tend to do so because of embarrassment about communicating needs, mixed messages, reduced self-confidence and unrealistic expectations about what 'the norm' is regarding sex. All these, and others, can relate to both partners. Although changes may need to be made to your sex life, it is still possible for both of you to have a fulfilling sex life.

17

Nights are the worst time

➔ Key Points

◆ People often have unrealistic expectations about how much sleep they need and what is a normal sleep pattern

◆ There are no set number of hours that people should be sleeping for. We need to judge how much sleep we need by whether we are coping with things the next day

◆ A graph of a normal sleep pattern would look more like an up and down rollercoaster than a U shape. When we sleep, we do not fall into a deep sleep and remain at that depth until the next morning. The depth of our sleep fluctuates throughout the night and there are times during the night when we sleep very lightly and sometimes wake up, but we may not remember this

◆ There are things that people do that they think will help their situation but they may make the problem worse

◆ There are things that people can do that will help them to sleep better

Sleep problems are extremely common in people with pain. The problem may be finding it hard to get to sleep, waking up through the night or not being able to return to sleep after waking up. Poor sleep can result in feeling slowed mentally and physically, being less able to enjoy things, feeling irritable or low in mood and people often say that their pain is often harder to cope with during these days.

📄 Case study

Ms Davis is 39 years old and has had back pain for five years. She stopped working over a year ago because she felt unable to continue working with her back pain. She feels very unmotivated and misses the structure that she used to have at work. Ms Davis now spends much of her day pottering around her flat and watching television. Although she has tried to do more during the day this just increases her pain. She sleeps for an hour during the day, most days, to escape her pain. She dreads bedtime because she finds it hard to sleep and when she eventually gets to sleep the pain wakes her up. She therefore avoids going to bed until after 2 o'clock in the morning. Ms Davis thinks she should be getting at least seven hours sleep a night and spends much of the night worrying about how little sleep she is getting. She sleeps until late morning and then feels frustrated because she has missed half of the day.

So what can you do to help improve your sleep? The first important thing to think about is whether you know, or what you think a 'normal' night's sleep is. Ask yourself these questions:

+ How many hours should people sleep for a night?
+ What is a normal sleep pattern (for example, is it normal to go to sleep, fall deeper asleep and stay like this until you awake next morning)?
+ What is helpful and unhelpful when people are having problems sleeping?

The reason it is important to ask yourself and find out the answer to these questions is that if you have unrealistic expectations about how you 'should' be sleeping then it is unlikely that you will achieve your goal. This may lead to increased frustration with your sleep, and frustration will only make the problem worse.

How many hours should people sleep for a night?

There are many research studies about sleep and how long we should sleep for. Many conclude that, on average, we need seven to eight hours a night. However, this is an *average* and is not something that we all need to try and reach. There are some people who need less and some who need more. It is important not to focus too much on how many hours sleep you are getting. A more helpful guide is to think about whether the amount of sleep you are getting is enabling you to do what you need to and would like to do the next day. Many people answer 'no' straight away to this, but again it is important to remember that the majority of people with or without pain have some bad nights sleep and find the next day hard because they are tired, so it is normal to feel tired some days and if you expect yourself never to feel tired then you will be disappointed.

The amount of sleep we need varies according to age, gender, physical and emotional health, lifestyle, work and social demands. As we get older we need less sleep and have more wakeful periods through the night. Comparing your own sleep with others is not a useful guide.

What is a normal sleep pattern?

Many people believe that a normal sleep pattern is to gradually fall into a deep sleep and then stay like this until the morning when we gradually come out of our deep sleep (see Figure 17.1).

A normal sleep pattern is divided up into stages which is partly characterized by the depth of sleep. One sleep cycle has five stages in it and people tend to go through four to five sleep cycles a night. When sleep is plotted on a graph it would look much more like a rollercoaster than a U shape (see Figure 17.2).

There is no doubt that having long-term pain can lead to sleep problems. However, once people know that it is normal to come into a very light sleep during the night and to sometimes wake up at this point, this helps them to develop realistic expectations about their sleep and to worry less about waking up and therefore find it easier to get back to sleep.

What is helpful and unhelpful when people are having problems sleeping?

People try different things to help them deal with sleep problems. These may include tablets, alcohol, staying in bed for as long as possible just in case they fall asleep, or sleeping during the day. However, these may help at the beginning, but after a while they can lose their effectiveness and may even contribute to sleep problems.

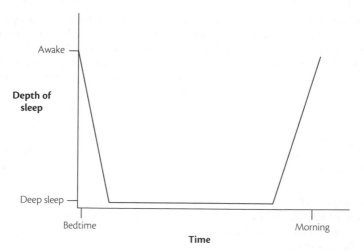

Figure 17.1 An unrealistic sleep pattern. This is not normal: do not expect this to happen.

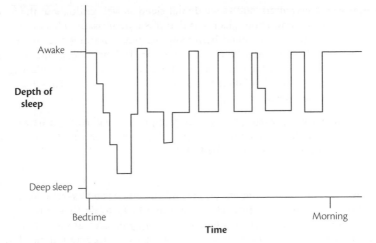

Figure 17.2 A normal sleep pattern.

Think about what the sleep problems you have are and what you have tried to do about them—try not to think, 'Oh, I've tried that before, it doesn't work.' It may be that you need to try it for longer and/or that it will help in combination with something else.

Food and drink

It is important to think about what you eat and drink in the night if you wake up but also a few hours before you go to bed because things can stay in your body for longer than you may think.

Stimulants do just that. They stimulate us and keep us awake. Caffeine is a stimulant and is in many things that you may not be aware of. It can be found in coffee, tea, chocolate, cola drinks, green tea, and even some painkillers. Try to avoid drink and food with caffeine four to six hours before bed time as this will give the caffeine a chance to stop stimulating your body. If you wake up at night and are someone who is comforted by a hot drink, then again avoid stimulating ones. Try drinking warm milk or a herbal tea (but check the packaging as some of these contain caffeine). The nicotine in cigarettes is also a stimulant, yet having a cigarette is something that people often do in the middle of the night when they cannot sleep. Try to avoid this because you need to prevent your body from being stimulated during the night.

You may be one of the many people who drink alcohol to help them sleep. However, alcohol is one of the things that may help you to get to sleep but then it causes other difficulties. Although you may get to sleep easily, alcohol tends to make us wake up earlier in the morning and so we get less sleep. It also disrupts our sleep pattern and so we do not sleep as well throughout the night. Another thing to know about alcohol is that it is a depressant. This means that it may contribute to your mood being low the next morning and, of course, if you are already someone who feels low and tired, then alcohol will make the situation more difficult for you. It is for these reasons that we would suggest trying to keep your alcohol intake low and do not use it on a nightly basis as a means to help you sleep.

Feeling hungry will prevent you from sleeping but so will eating a heavy meal close to bedtime. If you feel hungry before going to bed then have a light snack. Avoid eating heavy meals near to bedtime.

Exercise and stretch

We have already stressed the importance of movement and exercise for people who have back pain. However, choose a time of day to do these that is good for you. Aerobic exercise during the day will help you sleep at night. However, because exercise stimulates us, it can prevent us from sleeping if done close to bedtime.

Gentle stretching should not keep you awake, in fact it might help you to sleep. Some people find it helpful to stretch before going to bed and when they wake up in the night they stretch in bed or get out of bed for a short period and stretch.

Routine

Many people recognize the importance of routine to help a baby to sleep, but for some reason we forget that this can also be helpful for adults. Having a regular 'wind down time' for about an hour before you go to bed will help you and your body to prepare mentally and physically for sleep. For example, you might turn off the television, have a warm bath (not too hot because our bodies like to cool down slightly to be able to go to sleep), have a warm drink, do some relaxation or stretches. Make this a habit and follow the same sequence every night.

It is also important to have a routine in terms of when you go to bed and get up.

Get up at the same time every morning, no matter how well or badly you slept the night before. Some people may think that it is a good idea to stay in bed for a little longer to try and catch up on sleep. However, this is not helpful as the sleep that you get during this period will not be very refreshing, it stops you from sticking to a set time to get up and it will encourage you to go to bed later that evening.

Go to bed when you are sleepy because you are more likely to fall asleep rather than toss and turn.

Daytime sleeping

If you have problems sleeping at night try not to sleep even for a short time during the day, no matter how tired you feel. If you find yourself dozing during the day do something that will stop you from falling asleep. For example, go for a walk, do some exercise, visit a friend. Keeping sleep for night time helps your body and mind to make a clear distinction between day and night.

Some people's pattern of sleeping is back to front: they tend to spend a lot of the night up and awake and a lot of the day in bed asleep. This is often a pattern that has built up over time. Although initially it may seem to help because at least you are sleeping, there are enormous disadvantages to this, not least because you are missing out on a lot of life and interactions with other people and normal working hours become impossible. If you recognize this in yourself and would like to change this pattern, it is important to change this habit gradually. So, for example, if you normally go to bed at 4 o'clock in the morning and get up at 1 o'clock in the afternoon, try going to bed 15 minutes earlier and get up 15 minutes earlier. Then gradually push the time you go to bed and get up earlier by 15 minutes each day, every other day or each week, whatever suits you.

Your bedroom

It is important to help your mind associate your bedroom and bed with sleep. Therefore keep your bedroom just for sleep and sex. Remove televisions, computers, telephones and desks from your bedroom. Try not to use your bedroom during the day and do not work in your bedroom. Obviously that can be hard for some people depending on their living situation. If you have to work in your bedroom then try to make an area that is just for work as far away from your bed as you can and separate it from the rest of your room with something like a screen.

Make your bedroom as dark as possible so that you are not woken by light when you are in one of your lighter sleeping periods. It can be helpful to have a window open because a well-ventilated room can aid sleep.

Not being able to get to sleep or waking up in the night

If you find that you have not gone to sleep after about 15–20 minutes then get up: you want to avoid your body and mind associating your bed with being awake. Go to another room (for the same reason) and do something restful or monotonous until you feel sleepy again, then return to bed. Stretches and relaxation exercise may help you at this time. Do not do something like watch an exciting film or a read an exciting book because these will stimulate your mind and reduce the chances of you returning to sleep.

If you wake up at night, do not look at the clock: finding out the time will probably irritate you. If there is a long way to the morning you might become frustrated or anxious because you hate the thought of being in bed and not sleeping for all those hours that are ahead of you. If there is only a short time before the morning you may get quite anxious because you are desperate to have more sleep. Put the clock in a drawer or turn it round so you cannot see the face but make sure you will be able to hear the alarm if you need to get up at a certain time.

Thoughts, feeling and sleeplessness

As we discussed in Chapter 8, our thoughts, feelings and behaviour all influence each other. If we take sleep as the behaviour, this is no exception. Being flooded by unhelpful thoughts during the night will get in the way of sleep. Common unhelpful thoughts are:

◆ 'I should be getting more sleep than this.'

◆ 'There's no way I'll be able to cope with tomorrow if I don't sleep.'

◆ 'I'll never be able to get to sleep.'

When you become aware of unhelpful thoughts about a potential lack of sleep, try and challenge them. Examples of challenges are:

◆ 'It won't help if I put pressure on myself to sleep. There is no "should" about how many hours of sleep I should be getting. Some sleep is better than none.'

◆ 'I've been tired many times before and although these days haven't been plain sailing, I've always been able to achieve something. There have never been days when I've done absolutely nothing.'

◆ 'Telling myself I'll never sleep will make it more unlikely that I'll fall asleep. Even if I rest it's better that being restless and worried.'

Worrying at night about things in your life will also keep you awake. People often say that they lie awake at night worrying about their pain, their family, their financial situation, work, deadlines that they are trying to reach and their future. If you tend to do this, the following can be helpful.

◆ At least two hours before bedtime give yourself some time to write down your worries and what you plan to do about them the next day. If you wake up in the night, remind yourself that you have given these some time already, that going over it now will not help and that you can think about it the next day.

◆ Keep a pad of paper by your bed. If you wake up worrying about something that you did not address during your 'worry time', then write it down on the paper and tell yourself that you'll give it time tomorrow but now it is time to sleep.

◆ Imagery can help some people push away their worries at night. For example, you might find it helpful to imagine putting your worries in boxes that are hanging from a pulley system and then pushing them away from you. Or placing your worries in a boat that drifts away from you.

Just like Ms Davis, many people dread going to bed and have an association in their mind between their bedroom/bed and sleepless nights, distress, frustration and so on. Not only is it important to try practical strategies to change this association, but it will be helpful if you become aware of and challenge the unhelpful thoughts that lead to a feeling of dread before you go to bed. These thoughts may be something like:

- 'I just know tonight will be as bad as all the other.'
- 'I hate my bedroom. It's the worst place in my flat. It'll always be like this.'

And finally...

If you do not sleep well and decide to try some of the above, we would recommend trying one or two things at a time and no more. Give yourself and your body time to adapt to these one or two changes and when you do, then you can try another. It is important that your expectations about how effective these will be are realistic. It may take time for you to notice any improvements: some will be harder than others, and some will be more helpful than others.

18

My pain has got a whole lot worse

➡️ Key Points

- Sometimes it is obvious what has caused in increase in pain. Sometimes it is hard to find out. The nature of long-term pain is that it can increase without warning

- Although this time can be unpleasant, if you incorporate the pain management techniques that are discussed in this book in a 'flare-up plan', this will help you during these times

- A flare-up plan is not about reducing your pain level. It is a plan to help you manage this difficult time and to help you maintain some movement and activity rather than the pain stopping you in your tracks

📄 Case study

Mr Grey is 60 years old and has had back pain for three years. His pain is constant but there are times when it increases in severity. Sometimes he can say why this happens, sometimes he has no idea. During these times Mr Grey feels that he cannot move, his mood is very low and he feels frustrated. When his pain begins to increase he goes to bed or lies on his sofa and takes the maximum amount of pain medication that he can in the hope that he will sleep. When this does not help, Mr Grey calls an ambulance or asks his neighbour to take him to casualty. In casualty they give him an injection which sometimes reduces his pain a little and then they send him home. Mr Grey then spends three to five days in bed until he feels able to walk again.

What causes an increase in my pain?

Everyone's back pain can vary in intensity or severity, and there will be some days when your back hurts more than other days. Although it can be a difficult time, this fluctuation in pain is totally normal and is often called a 'flare-up' in pain. Just like Mr Grey, sometimes it is possible to recognize what has caused a flare-up. The causes can include:

◆ Overdoing an activity, for example, doing something for too long or carrying something that is heavier than your carrying tolerance (see Chapter 12)

◆ Resting for too long (or staying in the same position for too long)

◆ Not taking enough short breaks.

It may be helpful to remember that some flare-ups can be caused by something someone did a few days ago rather than on the day their pain increases. Therefore it may be helpful to think about what you have been doing over the last few days. However, it is worth remembering that flare-ups can also happen for no apparent reason.

> If you are unable to work out what may have caused your flare-up, then rather than dwell on this and give yourself a hard time, it is better to start thinking about how you can manage your flare-up.

When people have a flare-up they often do things that may help initially and in the short term. For example, it is understandable why Mr Grey believes that resting for a few days would help him. He may believe that an increase in pain is due to damage and therefore he believes he should rest to let the damage heal. However, we know that this is not necessarily the case, especially if the pain has been experienced for longer than three months. He might believe that the pain is telling him to stop and rest. Again when pain lasts longer than three months it is no longer an alarm—it is not actually telling us anything helpful.

In the long term things such as resting for long periods can lead to more problems. For example, many people go to bed for a few hours and take pain medication. This may help in the short term because they may feel a bit more relaxed and the medication may reduce the pain a little. However, as you may know, staying in one position for a long time (such as being in bed) can lead to stiffness and over a longer period of time muscles can become weak, all of which can result in more pain. Although a lot of people are tempted to rest during their flare-up, other people struggle on regardless and push themselves because they are determined not to let the flare-up get the better of them. However, this can result in a further increase in pain and a knock-on effect on their mood.

> The most important thing to remember is that an increase in your normal pain does not mean that you have done more damage.

I often go to casualty. What else can I do?

Some people can find this time so difficult that the only thing that they feel they can do is to go to casualty. It is understandable that people do this; they want someone to help them and to take the pain away. However, when asked if going to casualty helps, people often say that all that happened was that they were given an injection which did not really help and then they were sent home. If you think about what we have discussed about long-term pain, then this is not really surprising as there is nothing else the hospital staff can do. A flare-up is not caused by damage so there is little point in an X-ray or scan being done to try and find any damage. Long-term rest is not helpful even in a flare-up so there is little point in being admitted to hospital for bed rest. Although medication might be helpful in managing a flare-up, it would be better to discuss this with your local medical services. Going to casualty often involves waiting and a degree of anxiety which is not always helpful.

So what is the best thing to do when you have a flare-up? The strategies to use during this time are discussed throughout this book and are listed in the box below and then discussed in more detail.

Helpful strategies to use during a flare-up

- Challenging thoughts and feelings
- Pacing
- Planning and prioritizing
- Stretches and exercise
- Relaxation
- Helpful use of medication
- Developing and using a flare-up plan

Challenging thoughts and feelings

An increase in pain can affect people's mood. For example they can feel low, irritable, frustrated, worried, helpless and/or angry quite quickly. This can make it even harder to cope with a difficult time such as having a flare-up. As we discussed in Chapter 8, our thoughts, feelings, pain and what we do all affect each other (see Figure 8.4).

When you are having a flare-up, sooner rather than later it can be helpful to recognize the thoughts that are going through your mind because they will be influencing your emotions and how you cope with your flare-up. Common thoughts during a flare-up include:

◆ 'This is terrible, it'll never end.'
◆ 'I can't do anything today. I'll have to cancel all my plans.'
◆ 'I must have done more damage to myself.'

These thoughts can have an unhelpful effect on emotions:

Thought	Resulting emotion (or feeling)
'This is terrible, it'll never end.'	Depressed
'I can't do anything today. I'll have to cancel all my plans.'	Frustrated
'I must have done more damage to myself.'	Worry

They can also have an unhelpful effect on what you do during a flare-up:

Thought	Resulting emotion (or feeling)	What you do
'This is terrible, it'll never end.'	Depressed	Go to bed all day
'I can't do anything today. I'll have to cancel all my plans.'	Frustrated	Cancel meeting with friend. Spend the day on your own not doing anything enjoyable
'I must have done more damage to myself.'	Worry	Panic. Think about the pain all day and monitor if your pain gets worse.

These are just some examples. There are many other thoughts and emotions that you may have during a flare-up. All of these thoughts and emotions are understandable, although some may not be realistic. They are all unhelpful.

If you can manage to recognize yourself having thoughts like these, then it will help you to challenge them and replace them with different, more helpful thoughts. For example:

Unhelpful thought	More helpful thought
'This is terrible, it'll never end.'	'My pain has increased which may make my day harder, but there are things I can do so it doesn't feel too terrible. I've had flare-ups before and I've managed most of them quite well. The pain has always come down to its normal level.'
'I can't do anything today. I'll have to cancel all my plans.'	'Maybe there are some things I can do today. I don't have to cancel all my plans, just some of them. I'll still do one or two things I had planned but I'll give myself more time and do things more gently. I'll make sure that one of them is something I enjoy.'
'I must have done more damage to myself.'	'I remember being told that an increase in my pain doesn't mean that I've done more damage. I may have overdone things yesterday but I also know that flare-ups can happen for no apparent reason. Although it hurts, there's nothing to worry about. Rather than worrying about damage I need to think about how I manage this.'

See Chapter 8 for a more in-depth discussion on how to recognize and challenge unhelpful thoughts.

Pacing

It is very important to achieve a balance between resting too much and pushing yourself too much. During a flare-up it can be tempting to let your level of activity be guided by your pain, doing less on the days when you have a flare-up and more on a better day. However, this will lead to:

♦ The pain (rather than you) being in control of your activity level and what you do.

- You are more likely to be in the over/underactivity cycle which can lead to more difficulties (see Chapter 12).

- You will spend a period of time being quite inactive which means you will become stiffer and lose some fitness and so it will be harder to build up again (see Chapter 11).

- You may not achieve anything or do anything that you enjoy and this may lower your mood (see Chapter 8).

It is because of these points that pacing is essential (Chapter 12). This will prevent you from resting for too long or from overdoing an activity and will help you to achieve a balanced level of activity. Although it can be very tempting to reduce your tolerance levels it is important to keep to your tolerance levels during a flare-up. This is to help you remain in control rather than your pain and to prevent you from going back into the over/underactivity cycle. So for example, if you usually sit for ten minutes still try to do this when you have a flare-up. If you have gradually been increasing your tolerances, do not increase them any more until your flare-up has settled down and your pain is back to its usual level.

Planning and prioritizing

Using your pain management skills to help you during a flare-up does not mean stopping everything else that you had planned for the day. It is important that you think about what you had planned and prioritize the things that need doing or that you want to do. This may mean re-scheduling some things, but not everything. Stick to a few plans even if it means you change them slightly. For example, if you had planned to meet a friend in town, maybe arrange to meet them locally or in your home. Try and plan one or two enjoyable things to do during the day. Even though you may not gain as much enjoyment from them as you usually do, it may help to lift your mood a little.

Stretches and exercises

Stretches and exercises are important during these days even though you may not feel like doing them. This is because it is important to maintain a gentle level of activity each day (see Chapter 12). Just like Mr Grey many people feel that they cannot move the painful parts of their body on these days. However, if you begin by gently stretching the less painful areas of your body you may find that you can then begin to gently stretch the more painful areas. When you stretch on these days, follow the principles listed in the box below.

> ### Principles of stretching during a flare-up
> - Gently
> - Slowly

♦ Little

♦ Often

You will probably find that the range of your stretch (how far you can stretch) will be less when you have a flare-up. This is normal. Rather than pushing to achieve the range that you manage on a better day, just stretch to as far as is comfortable without causing more pain. Rather that doing your stretches all at once (as you may do on a better day) you may find it helpful to follow the principle of 'little and often' and spread them out over the day.

Relaxation

Relaxation can be helpful when you have a flare-up. When pain increases your body may become tense and you may find that you are breathing in your upper chest rather than down near your abdomen. Relaxation does not have to be about lying down for a long time. This can be hard during a flare-up. Using relaxation skills for even two to three minutes can be useful. See Chapter 10 to read about some relaxation techniques. There are a few things that may be helpful to remember when you practice relaxation during a flare-up:

♦ Use short rather than long relaxation techniques during a flare-up—for example, abdominal breathing and body scan (see Chapter 10).

♦ Practise these techniques little and often throughout the day.

♦ Don't expect too much of yourself when you are trying to relax during a flare-up. It will be harder to do during these times so do not expect to be able to relax as well as you can do on a better day.

Medication

It varies between people as to whether medication can be helpful during a flare-up. Some people find that the negatives of any side effects outweigh the benefits of pain relief and others find that they do not get any pain relief from medication. Even if you do use medication to manage a flare-up it is important to use the strategies that are outlined in this section. It is also important to follow the guidelines in the box below.

Medication guidelines for a flare-up

♦ Make sure you take no more than the recommended dose.

♦ Take your medication at regular time intervals, as prescribed or as written on the box/bottle, rather than taking it all at once or trying not to take it until your pain is unbearable.

◆ Have a plan to reduce your medication back to its usual level within about seven days (or to have stopped your medication if you were not taking it before). Plan a gradual reduction rather than suddenly going back down to the amount that you were taking before your flare-up. For example, if you take two tablets four times a day for the first two days, you may decide to take two tablets three times a day for the next two days, then two tablets twice a day for the next two days, then one tablet twice a day for one day, and then stop them the next day.

Flare-up plan

Concentrating and planning can be hard during a flare-up. This makes it even harder to decide what to do for the best. A pre-prepared flare-up plan can help to make a flare-up a little more manageable. A flare-up plan is a list that you write. It contains activities and pain management strategies that you find useful and helpful during a flare-up. It can be helpful to write down how many minutes you will do each activity for (see the example of a flare-up plan below). The aim of a flare-up plan is not to reduce your pain but to help you to manage your flare-up and rather than the pain stopping you in your tracks, to continue to do at least some of the activities that you had planned. In the box below there is a list of things that people have said can be helpful during a flare-up.

Examples of things that people have found helpful in a flare-up

◆ Stretching
◆ Having a cup of tea
◆ Using relaxation techniques
◆ Having a shower
◆ Taking a short rest
◆ Phoning a good friend
◆ Taking a warm bath
◆ Going for a short walk
◆ Gentle exercising
◆ Using a hot water bottle
◆ Using ice packs
◆ Watching a favourite film

This table is an example of a flare-up plan.

Activity or pain management strategy	Length of time I'll do it for
Check my thoughts and challenge any unhelpful thoughts that are making me panic and feel depressed	10 minutes
Gentle stretches whilst waiting for the kettle to boil to make a cup of tea	5 minutes
Focus on my breathing	5 minutes
After my cup of tea, go outside and walk down the street and back to my flat	10 minutes (4 minutes walk, 2 minutes rest, 4 minutes walk back to flat)
Gentle stretches	2 minutes
Phone Jane, Sarah or John and try and arrange something for later	10 minutes
Check my thoughts again	3 minutes
Watch 30 minutes of television but make sure I pace my sitting and standing. Stretch after 15 minutes	30 minutes
Scan my body for signs of tension	3 minutes
Work at my computer making sure I pace my sitting	20 minutes
Gentle exercises with a break halfway through	15 minutes

Prolonged flare-ups

A flare-up is an increase in pain that lasts anything from two hours to two days. If your pain increases for longer than two days we call this a prolonged flare-up. Everything written above will be helpful during a prolonged flare-up so it is important to keep trying all your pain management strategies.

There is one area where you may want to try something different. During a flare-up it is important to try to keep your tolerances (for example, your time for sitting) the same that they were the day before and not to be tempted to reduce them. During a prolonged flare-up it may be helpful to reduce your tolerances by about half. So for example if your standing tolerance is 10 minutes, cut this down to 5 minutes. If you had built up to carrying for 6 minutes, cut this back to 3 minutes. If you do this is it important that you have a plan to increase your tolerances back to where they were within about seven days. So, for the standing example:

Standing tolerance the day before my prolonged flare-up (Monday)	10 minutes
Standing tolerance the day my prolonged flare-up began (Tuesday)	5 minutes
Standing tolerance Wednesday	5 minutes
Standing tolerance Thursday	5 minutes 30 seconds
Standing tolerance Friday	6 minutes
Standing tolerance Saturday	7 minutes
Standing tolerance Sunday	8 minutes
Standing tolerance Monday	9 minutes
Standing tolerance Tuesday	10 minutes

Times of increased pain can be difficult. However, they will feel more manageable if you think about and apply the strategies discussed above. It is essential that you have realistic expectations about these strategies at this difficult time. They are to help you manage a flare-up rather than decrease your pain.

Appendix

Internet resources

Back care is a charity promoting and supporting healthier backs.

http://www.backcare.org.uk/

The British Pain Society has a webpage for patients with a number of links to other organizations with an interest in various aspects of pain, including back pain.

http://www.britishpainsociety.org.uk/

The NHS Clinical Knowledge Summaries (formerly PRODIGY) are a reliable source of evidence-based information and practical know-how about the common conditions managed in primary care. There are a lot of electronic pages of information for patients and the link below takes you to the section on back pain.

http://cks.library.nhs.uk/patient_information_leaflet/back_pain

Pain Concern is a charity that supplies information and support for pain sufferers, those who care for them and about them. They provide factsheets and leaflets to help you manage your pain as well as the 'Listening-ear helpline' which offers an opportunity to talk to another pain sufferer.

http://www.painconcern.org.uk/

Index